Published by Breastfeeding & Beyond Publishing
~Where evidence and tenderness belong together~

For permission requests, please contact:
Breastfeeding & Beyond
Bella Vista NSW, Australia
www.breastfeedingandbeyond.com.au

ISBN: 978-1-7643183-2-7

Cover design: Melody Jackson

Printed in Australia / Distributed worldwide via Amazon KDP

HEALING CONNECTIONS: HOW DEVELOPMENTAL TRAUMA INFLUENCES BREASTFEEDING RELATIONSHIPS

Dr Melody Jackson
Breastfeeding Medicine GP and IBCLC

ABOUT THE AUTHOR

Dr Melody Jackson is a Breastfeeding Medicine Physician, General Practitioner, International Board Certified Lactation Consultant (IBCLC), educator, and author based in Sydney, Australia. She is the Clinical Director of Breastfeeding & Beyond, where she supports families experiencing complex feeding, parenting, and perinatal mental health challenges.

Throughout her clinical work, Dr Jackson has developed a particular interest in the ways that developmental trauma, adverse childhood experiences, attachment, and neurobiology can influence breastfeeding relationships. Her work integrates evidence-based medicine with trauma-informed, relationship-centred care, helping clinicians and families better understand the emotional experiences that can accompany infant feeding.

Dr Jackson serves in leadership and educational roles within breastfeeding medicine both nationally and internationally. She is a board member of the Academy of Breastfeeding Medicine, an Adjunct Senior Clinical Lecturer at the University of Notre Dame Sydney School of Medicine, and a regular speaker on breastfeeding medicine, perinatal mental health, and trauma-informed care. She is also the author of her poetry collection, *Tender Thresholds: Reflections on Motherhood and Medicine*.

In *Healing Connections*, Dr Jackson brings together clinical experience, research evidence, and compassionate reflection to explore the often-overlooked intersection of developmental trauma and breastfeeding. Her goal is to help clinicians and families move beyond blame and self-judgement toward greater understanding, safety, and connection.

ACKNOWLEDGMENT OF COUNTRY

I acknowledge the Traditional Custodians of the land on which this work was written, the Bidjigal people of the Dharug Nation, and pay my deep respects to Elders past and present. I honour their enduring connection to land, water, sky, and community — connections that have held and sustained life for tens of thousands of years.

I recognise that this land holds both story and scar. It has witnessed care, connection, and continuity — but also disruption, dispossession, and intergenerational trauma. These histories are not separate from the present; they live on in bodies, in families, and in the systems that shape how care is given and received.

I recognise that this land has always been a place of birth, of feeding, of mothering, of loss, and of healing. Long before clinical language and systems of care, there were ways of knowing how to hold mothers and babies — ways grounded in relationship, rhythm, and deep listening.

I offer respect to the mothers, parents, and babies who have come before us, who come now, and who are yet to arrive. I acknowledge that experiences of feeding, care, and connection are shaped not only by the present moment, but by layers of lived and inherited experience, including trauma.

May this work be held with the same spirit of care — one that values safety, honours story, and makes space for healing.

PURPOSE AND TERMINOLOGY OF THIS BOOK

This resource aims to provide healthcare professionals with comprehensive knowledge, practical strategies, and compassionate approaches for supporting lactating parents who have experienced trauma. It explores developmental trauma, birth trauma, and complex trauma, and considers how these experiences may influence feeding relationships, attachment, identity, and wellbeing during the perinatal period.

Throughout this book, I use a range of terms when discussing parenting and infant feeding. At times, I may use words such as mother, woman, or maternal, particularly when discussing research, physiology, identity, or when reflecting the language used by individuals themselves. At other times, I may use more inclusive language such as parent, birthing parent, or lactating person to acknowledge the diversity of people who breastfeed, chestfeed, express milk, or nurture infants.

My intention is not to erase or diminish anyone's identity, but rather to create space for the many ways people experience parenting, feeding, bodies, and care.

Similarly, language used to describe people who have experienced trauma is often imperfect. Terms such as victim and survivor are widely used in clinical, research, legal, and advocacy settings. While these terms may feel empowering, validating, or personally meaningful for some individuals, they may not resonate with others.

Personally, I find that neither term fully captures the complexity of people's lives and experiences. Victim can at times emphasise what was done to a person, while survivor may unintentionally imply that healing, resilience, or recovery should look a certain way. Many people do not identify with either label, and some move between different understandings of their experiences over time.

For this reason, I generally prefer person-first language, such as people who have experienced trauma, people with a history of trauma, or simply individuals. However, because this book draws on research, clinical practice, lived experience narratives, and existing literature, a range of terminology may be used throughout. When such terms appear, they are not intended to define, limit, or categorise individuals, but rather to reflect the language used within a particular context.

I recognise that language in these areas can feel deeply personal and, at times, emotionally charged. I invite readers to approach these differences with curiosity, humility, and respect, while keeping our shared focus on compassionate, evidence-informed care for families.

CONTENT WARNING

We all bring our unique and complex lived experiences into our professional roles. This resource will cover topics that may be difficult or triggering, and I will be sharing stories, quotes, and reflections that may stir strong emotions, whether or not you have personal experience with them.

Just as I say when discussing these topics in “real life”, if this isn’t the right moment for you to engage, please honour your needs — put this guide down if necessary and return when you feel ready.

PROLOGUE: WHY THIS BOOK EXISTS

This book was born out of years of listening, witnessing, and walking alongside families navigating one of the most transformative and vulnerable experiences of their lives: breastfeeding and parenting after trauma. As a breastfeeding and lactation medicine (BFLM) physician, general practitioner and IBCLC, I have sat with mothers as they breastfed through tears, through grief, through past memories that surfaced in the most unexpected moments. I have held stories that cracked me open, stories I carry with reverence and responsibility.

Over time, I began to notice common threads. The quiet pauses. The words left unsaid. The body language that spoke louder than any history form. And I realised something: we cannot fully support breastfeeding families unless we understand trauma. Not just in theory, but in practice, in relationship, in language, in presence.

In *Healing Connections*, we explore the profound effects that developmental and other traumas can have on the breastfeeding journey. As a clinician and a passionate advocate for trauma-informed care, my goal is to integrate rigorous research with empathetic, real-world practice.

This resource is written for the clinician who wants to do better — not perfectly, but with more compassion, insight, and effectiveness. It is for the IBCLC, the doctor, the midwife, the nurse, the trainee, and the experienced practitioner who suspects there is more to the story and wants to know how to help without harming.

It is also written with deep gratitude for the mothers who have trusted me with their stories, who have spoken truths that the world often silences, and who have allowed their experiences to inform and inspire this work. I hope their voices echo throughout these pages.

Trauma does not mean breastfeeding must be abandoned. But it does mean we must tread gently. We must listen more deeply. And we must expand our definitions of success, healing, and connection.

Let this book be both a guide and a companion. You are not alone in this work. And neither are the families you serve.

TABLE OF CONTENTS

CHAPTER 1:

Understanding Trauma in the Perinatal Period

Trauma is not what happens to you,

it is what happens inside you as a result of

what happens to you.

~ Dr Gabor Mate

DEFINING TRAUMA AND ITS NUANCES

Trauma is not always visible. It does not always arrive with a label or a diagnosis. Sometimes it shows up in the silence, in the startle, in the tearful latch, in the refusal to be touched. As breastfeeding medicine providers, we must learn to see it.

WHAT IS TRAUMA?

Trauma is a person's emotional response to a distressing experience. It often overwhelms one's ability to cope and undermines a sense of safety in the world. Unlike ordinary hardship, trauma is sudden, unpredictable, and accompanied by a sense of helplessness or horror. The most important thing to understand is that trauma is defined not by the event itself, but by the individual's experience of it.[1]

Trauma is far more than a stressful event – it is a profound emotional wound that can alter the very fabric of one's sense of safety and self. Trauma often involves a disruption in one's core belief systems, shifting how the individual experiences control, intimacy, and trust. It is characterised by an overwhelming sense of vulnerability and unpredictability, leaving those who have experienced it feeling as though the threat might return at any moment.[2]

Trauma affects the body, brain, relationships, and behaviours. It can shape how a person views themselves, others, and the world around them. It can impact parenting, attachment, and the ability to seek or accept help, and it can profoundly influence the breastfeeding relationship.[2-4]

Recent qualitative research underscores that trauma in the perinatal period is frequently unspoken, unrecognised, and underestimated within healthcare settings. Women with histories of sexual trauma and interpersonal violence often do not disclose these experiences during pregnancy or postpartum care, yet their impact may emerge through heightened distress, loss of bodily autonomy, or difficulty tolerating touch and exposure.[5] These responses are not always recognised as trauma-related, particularly when clinicians rely on disclosure rather than observation.

A growing body of evidence highlights that perinatal trauma has enduring psychological effects, shaping emotional safety, trust in healthcare systems, and relational capacity well beyond the immediate event.[6] For many women, pregnancy and birth represent a convergence point where earlier trauma and current vulnerability intersect. Without trauma-informed awareness, clinicians may misinterpret survival responses as anxiety, resistance, or disengagement.

Importantly, clinicians themselves describe significant challenges in identifying and responding to trauma within routine perinatal care. An integrative review of midwifery practice found that while healthcare professionals recognise the importance of trauma-informed care, many feel undertrained and under-supported to initiate conversations about trauma safely.[7] This gap reinforces the need for universal, assumption-free approaches that prioritise emotional safety regardless of disclosure.

LAYERS OF TRAUMA: TIMING, REPETITION AND RELATIONSHIP

Not all trauma is the same. It's origins, durations and context shape how it is experienced and how it echoes into the future. As clinicians, recognising these distinctions helps us tailor our care and respond with the sensitivity required.[2]

1. Acute *(Single-Incident)* Trauma

These are events that occur suddenly and without warning. They are often isolated in time but carry the potential for lasting psychological and physiological impact.

Examples:
Car accidents, natural disasters, a one-time physical or sexual assault, an unexpected obstetric emergency.

Impact:
Even a single traumatic event can overwhelm the nervous system, shatter one's sense of safety, and leave behind hypervigilance, fear, and avoidance related to the triggering context.[1]

In perinatal care:
An emergency caesarean section or postpartum haemorrhage, even when medically well-managed, can become traumatic if the mother felt uninformed, powerless, or unsupported.[2]

2. Chronic *(Repeated or Ongoing)* Trauma

These traumas are experienced repeatedly over time, often in the context of relationships or environments that are supposed to provide safety.

Examples:
Ongoing domestic violence, extended NICU stays, repeated medical procedures without consent, systemic discrimination including racism.[3, 4]

Impact:
The cumulative nature of chronic trauma erodes self-trust, fosters a persistent sense of threat, and may result in emotional numbing or dissociation.

These individuals may appear "stoic" or disconnected, when in fact they are surviving.[2, 4]

In perinatal care:
Patients with a history of chronic trauma may struggle to advocate for

themselves, experience medical environments as threatening, or feel undeserving of support.[2]

3. Developmental *(Complex or Childhood)* Trauma

This trauma occurs during the most sensitive periods of development - often at the hands of caregivers - and becomes woven into a person's core sense of self and relational blueprint.[4]

Examples:
Childhood neglect, witnessing parental violence, separation from a primary caregiver, childhood physical, emotional or sexual abuse.[3]

Impact:
Because these events happen when the brain is still developing, they profoundly alter emotional regulation, attachment patterns, and neurobiological systems. Survivors may experience persistent shame, difficulty trusting others and chronic dysregulation. [3, 4]

In perinatal care:
These patients may have complex relationships with their bodies, struggle with feelings of worthlessness, and be highly sensitive to bodily exposure or touch. The breastfeeding journey can bring opportunities for healing - or be a source of distress - depending on the support offered.[2]

Single-incident trauma, particularly if experienced in adulthood, can be vastly different in its psychological and developmental impact than trauma experienced in early childhood. Developmental trauma - chronic exposure to relational and environmental harm in early life - shapes the architecture of the nervous system, sense of self, and relational worldview.[3, 4]

Trauma is not uniform. Its effects are deeply shaped by the developmental stage at which it occurs, the duration of exposure, and the resources or protective relationships available at the time. What overwhelms a 30-year-old may be very different from what overwhelms a 16-year-old or what overwhelms a 2-year-old. Context matters.[3]

In developmental trauma, the attachment relationship – often with the primary caregiver – is where the trauma originates or is compounded. This disrupts the development of a coherent self, a predictable world, and a safe way of being in relationship with others. Children do not have the same capacity to understand or verbalise their experiences. If trauma occurs before a child has developed a stable sense of self, it may leave them without an internal roadmap of who they are. These early maps of the world, encoded in the body and brain, are remarkably stable across time.[4]

Children who experience multiple, repeated traumas often suffer disruptions in emotional regulation, learning, memory, social functioning, and physical health. Their nervous systems may become wired to detect threat everywhere, making it difficult to distinguish real danger from perceived danger. They remain in survival mode – hyperalert, withdrawn, reactive – rather than feeling safe enough to explore, learn, and connect.[3, 4]

The effects of these patterns may persist into adulthood, manifesting as anxiety, difficulty in relationships, emotional dysregulation, and somatic symptoms. Even if the trauma occurred decades ago, the patterns it established can influence how a person navigates pregnancy, birth, and breastfeeding.[2, 4]

Experiences in pregnancy or the first four years of life may not be consciously remembered. However, research has shown that these early life experiences have significant, long-lasting impacts on neurodevelopment, attachment patterns, and emotional wellbeing.[3, 4] As Bessel van der Kolk writes: "the body keeps the score."[4] Even when the conscious mind cannot retrieve the memory, the body may hold the imprint.

This can be confusing for the traumatised person. They may struggle to understand why pregnancy or birth feels triggering, overwhelming, or shameful – especially when it is "supposed" to be a joyful time. When we recognise that trauma can be preverbal, invisible, and deeply embedded, we are better equipped to respond with empathy.[2]

Finally, it is important to acknowledge that trauma often begets trauma. Once someone has experienced a traumatic event, they are statistically more likely to encounter additional traumas in their lifetime. This makes trauma survivors – especially those with a history of developmental trauma – particularly vulnerable during the perinatal period.[3]

RECOGNISING TRAUMA RESPONSES: PATTERNS OF SURVIVAL

Trauma leaves its imprint not only on memory, but on the body, emotions, and behaviours. Survivors may not always have a formal diagnosis, but they often live with persistent symptoms that reflect the nervous system's attempts to protect them from future harm. These responses are not signs of weakness – they are evidence of survival.[1, 2]

Intrusive Memories

These may include flashbacks, nightmares, or sudden, vivid recollections of past events. The trauma feels as though it is happening again in real time, often triggered by sensory reminders like smells, sounds, or touch.[1]

In the perinatal period, certain clinical procedures, baby cues, or even the act of breastfeeding itself may stir these memories, catching both parent and clinician off guard.

Avoidance

Avoidance can be subtle or overt. Survivors may steer clear of people, places, conversations, or even internal thoughts that remind them of the trauma. In a clinical setting, this might look like missed appointments, a reluctance to answer questions, or withdrawing emotionally during care. While often misunderstood as disinterest or noncompliance, avoidance is usually a protective strategy to prevent being retraumatised.[1, 2]

Negative Alterations in Mood and Cognition

These include persistent negative beliefs about oneself ("I'm broken," "I'm a bad mother"), emotional numbness, guilt, shame, mistrust of others, or a disconnection from loved ones. This detachment can interfere with the bonding process, making it difficult for parents to feel close to their baby or to receive support from others.[1, 2]

Hyperarousal and Reactivity

This refers to an increased state of physiological and emotional alertness. Survivors may startle easily, have difficulty sleeping, experience irritability or anger outbursts, or report physical tension that never quite resolves. These symptoms often lead to exhaustion, both physical and emotional, and can be especially challenging in the sleep-deprived early postpartum months.[1]

Hypervigilance: A Common but Overlooked Pattern

Hypervigilance is one of the most pervasive and under-recognised trauma responses, particularly during the perinatal period. It describes a sustained state of heightened alertness in which a person is constantly scanning for danger – both in their environment and within their own body or mind.

A helpful analogy is that of a smoke alarm that's become overly sensitive: it doesn't just activate when there's a real fire – it goes off when toast burns or the oven gets too hot. The system is working as intended: to keep the person safe, but the threshold has been lowered, and now the alarm is responding to cues that aren't actually dangerous.

In day-to-day life, hypervigilance may present as anxiety, restlessness, difficulty relaxing, irritability, or a strong need for control. For some, it shows up outwardly – checking on the baby constantly, over-preparing, or scanning for mistakes or potential harms. For others, it is more internal – a mental rehearsal of worst-case scenarios, or tightly managing routines to avoid feeling exposed or overwhelmed.

In new parents who have experienced trauma, hypervigilance can significantly impact bonding, feeding, and their own emotional recovery. They may feel "on edge" even in safe and loving environments. This heightened sensitivity is often misread as overanxious parenting or perfectionism, when in fact, it reflects a nervous system doing its best to protect what matters most.

Understanding hypervigilance as an adaptive, protective mechanism – one that has simply become overactive – can shift our perspective from judgment to compassion. It reminds us that these symptoms are not personal flaws but part of a body and mind doing the very best it can to feel safe again.

One mother described her experience vividly:

"I did get 'flashes' when I was feeding my baby.
Feeling gross and weird.
Feeling uncomfortable about my bodily autonomy in that this is my body and someone wants access to it you know?
Not just wanting access even, but worse, seeing my body as their own.
So I got very intrusive thoughts also not just around breastfeeding but just everything. Life.
It was severe for the first couple of weeks."

CLINICAL NOTE: DSM-5 CRITERIA FOR POST-TRAUMATIC STRESS DISORDER

The following diagnostic criteria are drawn from the Diagnostic and Statistical Manual of Mental Disorders, Fifth Edition (DSM-5), published by the American Psychiatric Association.[1]

In terms of a clinical diagnosis, to meet the diagnostic threshold for PTSD, an individual must have been exposed to actual or threatened death, serious injury, or sexual violence in one (or more) of the following ways:

- Directly experiencing the traumatic event(s)
- Witnessing the event(s) in person
- Learning that the traumatic event(s) occurred to a close family member or friend
- Experiencing repeated or extreme exposure to aversive details of traumatic events (e.g. first responders)

The individual must then exhibit symptoms from each of the following categories:

DSM-5 PTSD DIAGNOSTIC CRITERIA

Criterion A Exposure to Trauma	**Criterion B** Intrusion Symptoms
Criterion C Avoidance	**Criterion D** Negative Changes in Cognition and Mood
Criterion E Alterations in Arousal and Reactivity	**Criterion F** Duration
Criterion G Functional Impairment	**Criterion H** Exclusion

Source: American Psychiatric Association. DSM-5-TR (2022).

DSM-5 CRITERIA FOR POSTTRAUMATIC STRESS DISORDER (PTSD)

Exposure to actual or threatened death, serious injury, or sexual violence in one (or more) of the following ways:

Directly experiencing the traumatic event	Witnessing the event as it occurred to others	Learning that the event occurred to a close family member or close friend	Repeated or extreme exposure to aversive details of the event (e.g. first responders)

A

A. TRAUMATIC EXPOSURE
The individual was exposed to actual or threatened death, serious injury, or sexual violence in one (or more) of the ways above.

B

B. INTRUSION SYMPTOMS
One (or more) of the following associated with the traumatic event began after the event:

- Recurrent, involuntary, and intrusive distressing memories
- Distressing dreams
- Dissociative reactions (e.g. flashbacks)
- Intense or prolonged psychological distress at cues
- Marked physiological reactions to cues

C

C. AVOIDANCE
Persistent avoidance of stimuli associated with the traumatic event, beginning after the event, as evidenced by one (or both) of the following:

- Avoidance of distressing memories, thoughts, or feelings
- Avoidance of external reminders that arouse distressing memories, thoughts, or feelings

D

D. NEGATIVE ALTERATIONS IN COGNITIONS AND MOOD
Two (or more) of the following began or worsened after the event:

- Inability to remember important aspects of the event
- Persistent and exaggerated negative beliefs or expectations
- Blame of self or others
- Persistent negative emotional state (e.g. fear, horror, anger, guilt)
- Markedly diminished interest or participation in activities
- Feelings of detachment or estrangement
- Inability to experience positive emotions

E

E. ALTERATIONS IN AROUSAL AND REACTIVITY
Two (or more) of the following began or worsened after the event:

- Irritable behaviour and angry outbursts
- Reckless or self-destructive behaviour
- Hypervigilance
- Exaggerated startle response
- Problems with concentration
- Sleep disturbance

F.

F. DURATION
Duration of the disturbance is more than 1 month.

G.

G. CLINICALLY SIGNIFICANT DISTRESS OR IMPAIRMENT
The disturbance causes clinically significant distress or impairment in social, occupational, or other important areas of functioning.

H.

H. NOT DUE TO SUBSTANCE OR MEDICAL CONDITION
The disturbance is not attributable to the physiological effects of a substance or another medical condition.

Source: American Psychiatric Association. Diagnostic and Statistical Manual of Mental Disorders, 5th ed. (DSM-5®). Arlington, VA: APA; 2013.

Author note: While not all trauma survivors meet DSM criteria for PTSD, many will have subthreshold symptoms that still impact their parenting, breastfeeding, and mental health. Using trauma-informed principles helps us care for both groups with the same gentleness and skill.[2]

RECOGNISING TRAUMA RESPONSES: PATTERNS OF SURVIVAL

Trauma is far more common than many clinicians realise, and its effects often extend well beyond the original event. Rather than existing solely as a memory, trauma may influence how individuals perceive safety, respond to stress, experience relationships, and navigate the profound transitions of pregnancy, birth, and early parenthood. These responses are not signs of weakness or dysfunction; they are often adaptive strategies developed in the context of overwhelming experiences.

The perinatal period can bring both vulnerability and opportunity. Experiences of bodily change, dependency, intimacy, loss of control, and heightened responsibility may activate old patterns of coping, while new relationships with infants can also create possibilities for healing, growth, and reconnection. Understanding trauma through this lens shifts our focus from asking, "What is wrong with this parent?" to asking, "What has this parent experienced, and how might those experiences be influencing the present moment?"

For clinicians working in breastfeeding and infant feeding care, this perspective invites curiosity, compassion, and humility. Symptoms, behaviours, and feeding challenges that may initially appear puzzling often make sense when viewed within the context of a person's history and lived experience. Trauma-informed care begins not with specialised interventions, but with a willingness to recognise the impact of adversity and to create environments that promote safety, choice, collaboration, trust, and empowerment.

In the chapters that follow, we will explore how early adversity shapes development across the lifespan, beginning with the landmark Adverse Childhood Experiences (ACE) Study and its implications for health, parenting, and infant feeding. Understanding these foundations provides an important framework for recognising the many ways that past experiences can continue to influence the transition to parenthood.

REFERENCES

1 Association AP. Diagnostic and statistical manual of mental disorders. 5th edition ed. Arlington (VA): American Psychiatric Publishing; 2013.

2 Kimberg L, Wheeler M. Trauma and Trauma-Informed Care. 2019. p. 25–56.

3 Felitti VJ, Anda RF, Nordenberg D, Williamson DF, Spitz AM, Edwards V, et al. Relationship of childhood abuse and household dysfunction to many of the leading causes of death in adults. The Adverse Childhood Experiences (ACE) Study. Am J Prev Med. 1998;14(4):245–58.

4 Kolk vd. The body keeps the score: brain, mind, and body in the healing of trauma. New York: Viking; 2014.

5 Sobel L, O'Rourke-Suchoff D, Holland E, Remis K, Resnick K, Perkins R, et al. Pregnancy and Childbirth After Sexual Trauma: Patient Perspectives and Care Preferences. Obstet Gynecol. 2018;132(6):1461–8.

6 Perera E, Chou S, Cousins N, Mota N, Reynolds K. Women's experiences of trauma, the psychosocial impact and health service needs during the perinatal period. BMC Pregnancy Childbirth. 2023;23(1):197.

7 Callanan F, Bradshaw C, Tuohy T, Noonan M, Murphy S, Grealish A. An integrative review of how midwives are screening and assessing for trauma in women within perinatal services. PLoS One. 2025;20(7):e0327253.

CHAPTER 2:

The Study of Adverse Childhood Experiences (ACEs) and the Landscape of Early Adversity

"Adverse childhood experiences are the single greatest unaddressed public health threat facing our nation today."

~ Dr Robert Block

THE LANDMARK ACE STUDY: METHODOLOGY AND FINDINGS

The Adverse Childhood Experiences (ACE) study was a landmark investigation that first illuminated the profound relationship between early childhood adversity and later-life health outcomes. Conducted in the 1990s with more than 17 000 adult participants enrolled in the Kaiser Permanente health system in the United States, the study demonstrated that experiences such as abuse, neglect, and household dysfunction were not isolated events, but powerful determinants of long-term physical and mental health.[3]

As the number of adverse experiences increased, so too did the risk of a wide range of health conditions – including cardiovascular disease, diabetes, chronic lung disease, depression, substance use, and early mortality.[3] This clear dose–response relationship underscored the cumulative impact of trauma, showing that early adversity can alter stress physiology and biological systems in ways that predispose individuals to lifelong vulnerability.

The original ACE study identified ten categories of adverse childhood experiences, grouped into three broad domains:

Abuse
- Emotional abuse
- Physical abuse
- Sexual abuse

Neglect
- Emotional neglect
- Physical neglect

Household Dysfunction
- Exposure to domestic violence
- Household substance use

- Household mental illness
- Parental separation or divorce
- Incarcerated household member

Each exposure contributes one point to an individual's ACE score, with higher scores reflecting a greater cumulative burden of adversity. Importantly, the ACE framework is not a diagnostic tool. Rather, it offers a population-level lens through which to understand risk, resilience, and long-term health trajectories.[3]

The prevalence of adversity revealed by the study was striking. Nearly two-thirds of participants reported at least one ACE, and more than one in five reported three or more ACEs.[3] These findings challenged assumptions about the rarity of childhood trauma and reframed it as a widespread public health issue.

The ACE study also introduced the now widely cited concept of a dose–response relationship: as the number of ACEs increases, so does the risk of adverse outcomes. These effects are not merely psychological. Early adversity has been shown to influence brain development, immune functioning, endocrine regulation, and inflammatory pathways. Trauma, quite literally, gets under the skin.[4]

Subsequent research has expanded on these findings, exploring the mechanisms through which early adversity shapes adult health. Neurobiological studies have demonstrated that childhood stress can result in long-lasting changes in brain structure and function, particularly in systems involved in stress regulation, threat detection, and emotional processing.[4] Later work has also broadened the scope of ACE research to include impacts on behaviour, relationships, and quality of life, reinforcing the importance of early intervention and supportive care.

Taken together, the ACE study and its successors have fundamentally reshaped our understanding of how early life experiences influence health across the lifespan. They provide a critical foundation for trauma-informed care and highlight the importance of prevention, early identification, and integrated support systems. For clinicians and public health professionals, these insights are a call to action: addressing childhood trauma is not only a matter of individual healing, but a cornerstone of population health.[3]

WHY THE ACE STUDY MATTERS IN PERINATAL CARE

The ACE study is not about pathology – it is about preparation. For breastfeeding medicine providers, its findings invite us to assume the possibility of trauma rather than waiting for disclosure. Most mothers will not volunteer a trauma history unless they feel deeply safe, and many will not consciously connect early life experiences with current struggles.

The perinatal period represents a time of heightened vulnerability. Pregnancy, birth, and infant feeding place extraordinary demands on the body and nervous system. For individuals with significant ACEs, this period may reactivate long-standing patterns of threat, hypervigilance, or emotional dysregulation. This can manifest as anxiety, fear of touch, emotional reactivity, or difficulty forming secure bonds with the infant. For some, breastfeeding becomes an unexpected site of emotional overwhelm.

Contemporary research confirms that the psychological effects of childhood adversity often resurface during pregnancy and the postpartum period, even in individuals with no prior mental health diagnosis. Survivors of interpersonal trauma describe this life stage as one in which earlier coping strategies may become insufficient, and trauma responses previously held at bay may re-emerge.[4] These reactions are shaped by physiological change, relational vulnerability, and increased bodily exposure, rather than by weakness or pathology.

Understanding ACEs helps clinicians recognise that these responses are not disproportionate, attention-seeking, or pathological. They are adaptive responses shaped by earlier environments where safety could not be assumed.

PREVALENCE OF ACES AMONG MOTHERS

Subsequent research has confirmed that ACEs are highly prevalent in perinatal populations. In a large US study of more than 6,000 pregnant individuals, exposure to childhood adversity was common and often severe.[8]

Reported rates included:

- Penetrative rape - 16%
- Contact sexual abuse before age 18 - 25%
- Parental substance use - 32%
- Physical abuse - 34%
- Parental depression or mental illness - 36%

These figures underscore a critical reality: trauma is not rare. It presents daily in perinatal care settings, often silently. Without an explicit trauma-informed lens, its influence may be missed or misunderstood.

THE LASTING IMPACTS OF ACES

The effects of early adversity frequently emerge subtly during pregnancy and the postpartum period. While a patient may not disclose a trauma history, symptoms may nonetheless speak loudly. Without appropriate context, these symptoms are at risk of being misinterpreted or pathologised.

Physical Health Impacts

High ACE scores are associated with increased risk of a wide range of physical health conditions, including:

- Migraines
- Chronic pain syndromes (such as fibromyalgia, pelvic pain, or breast pain)
- Gastrointestinal disorders
- Gynaecological conditions
- Autoimmune and metabolic disease[3]

In some trauma survivors, pain becomes the primary language of distress. A parent may present with persistent breast or nipple pain that does not respond to standard treatment and lacks a clear physiological explanation. In such cases, it is important to consider whether trauma-related pain amplification or lowered pain thresholds may be contributing.[3, 4]

Physiological Dysregulation

Chronic hyperarousal is a hallmark consequence of early adversity. Individuals with significant ACEs may experience persistent activation of the stress response system, involving catecholamines, cortisol, and hypothalamic–pituitary–adrenal axis dysregulation.[4]

Even in the absence of immediate danger, the body behaves as though threat is ongoing. This "always-on" stress state can disrupt sleep, impair immune function, and contribute to chronic inflammation.

Sleep disturbance is particularly relevant in the perinatal period. For trauma-affected mothers, sleep may already be fragile. Well-intentioned advice such as "getting someone else to take the baby overnight" may paradoxically increase anxiety if separation from the infant heightens the sense of threat rather than relieving it.

Behavioural Impacts

Trauma-shaped behavioural patterns may include:

- Disordered eating or elevated BMI (sometimes serving as protection against unwanted attention or emotional exposure)
- Substance use, often used as a coping mechanism
- High-risk sexual behaviour linked to boundary violations and impaired self-worth
- Sleep disruption and self-neglect
- Acute or chronic suicidal ideation

These behaviours are not indicators of poor judgment. They are survival strategies that once served an adaptive purpose.

Cognitive and Emotional Consequences

Some of the most enduring effects of early adversity are internal and invisible. Trauma survivors may carry deeply ingrained beliefs such as:

- "I don't deserve care."
- "I am a burden."
- "I shouldn't be here."

These beliefs can profoundly interfere with help-seeking and engagement in perinatal care. Shame and self-blame may intensify during birth and breastfeeding, where bodily exposure and vulnerability are unavoidable. Low self-efficacy is also common, particularly for those whose early attachment relationships were unstable or unsafe.

Mistrust and heightened sensitivity to rejection may lead individuals to anticipate harm rather than support. In clinical settings, this can appear as withdrawal, resistance, or disproportionate emotional responses to neutral interactions.

Social and Relational Effects

Insecure attachment patterns developed in childhood often persist into adulthood. This may manifest as:

- Co-dependence – reliance on others for emotional regulation
- Hyper-independence – avoidance of support due to fear of harm

Both patterns can complicate the transition to parenthood and make it difficult to seek or accept help at a time of heightened need.

Pregnancy and Infant Health Outcomes

The effects of adverse childhood experiences can also extend into pregnancy and the health of the next generation. A growing body of research demonstrates associations between maternal ACE exposure and a range of obstetric and infant outcomes. These associations are thought to arise through complex pathways involving chronic stress physiology, behavioural coping strategies, and social determinants of health. [9-11]

Individuals with higher ACE scores are more likely to experience:

- Preterm birth
- Low birth weight
- Hypertensive disorders of pregnancy
- Gestational diabetes
- Increased obstetric intervention
- Postpartum depression and anxiety [9-11]

Infants born to parents with high ACE exposure may also be at increased risk of altered stress reactivity, difficulties with emotional regulation, and later developmental challenges.[12, 13] These patterns are not inevitable, but they reflect the ways in which early adversity can shape physiological systems across the lifespan.

Chronic activation of the maternal stress response appears to be one pathway linking childhood adversity with pregnancy outcomes. Dysregulation of the hypothalamic–pituitary–adrenal axis, increased inflammatory signalling, and altered cortisol patterns have all been observed in individuals with high ACE scores. During pregnancy, these changes may influence placental function, foetal growth, and the timing of labour.[9, 10]

Importantly, these findings should never be interpreted deterministically. Many parents with histories of adversity experience healthy pregnancies and have thriving children. Protective factors — including safe relationships, supportive healthcare environments, and trauma-informed care — can significantly buffer these risks.[14, 15]

For clinicians, awareness of these associations reinforces the importance of sensitive, relational care during pregnancy and the postpartum period. When providers recognise the possible long reach of early adversity, they are better positioned to interpret symptoms compassionately and to create environments that support both maternal and infant wellbeing.[14]

A TRAUMA-INFORMED PATHWAY TO UNDERSTANDING FEEDING DISTRESS

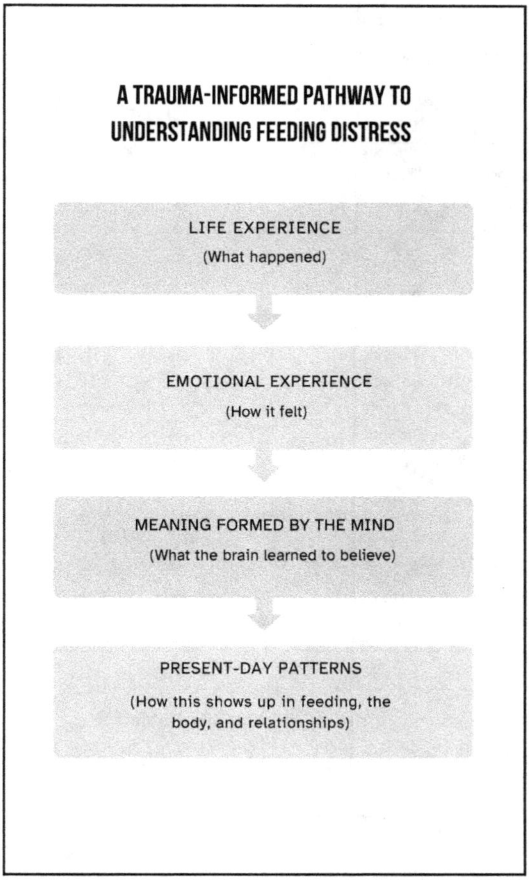

HOW TRAUMA SHAPES BELIEFS, BEHAVIOURS, AND FEEDING EXPERIENCES

EXPERIENCE	MEANING MADE AT THE TIME	CORE BELIEF THAT DEVELOPED	HOW IT MAY SHOW UP DURING FEEDING OR PARENTING
Traumatic birth, emergency surgery, medical crisis	"I was powerless"	"I am not safe in my body"	Hypervigilance, body tension, difficulty relaxing during feeds, fear when baby cries
Emotionally unavailable caregiver	"No one came when I needed them"	"I have to do everything alone"	Over-functioning, reluctance to ask for help, exhaustion
Childhood bullying or exclusion	"I don't belong"	"Something is wrong with me"	Shame, perfectionism, fear of 'getting feeding wrong'
Chronic criticism or microaggressions	"Mistakes are dangerous"	"I must not fail"	Anxiety, rigid expectations, distress when plans change
Sexual assault or boundary violation	"My body is not mine"	"Touch is unsafe"	Distress with latch, dissociation, discomfort with physical closeness
Unexpected loss, illness, divorce	"The world can change suddenly"	"The world is not safe or predictable"	Need for control, difficulty tolerating infant unpredictability
Pandemic, accident, or medical trauma	"I had to shut down to cope"	"Feelings are overwhelming"	Emotional numbing, detachment from feeding experience
Repeated relational rupture	"I cannot trust others"	"I must stay guarded"	Difficulty bonding, relational disconnection
High responsibility in childhood	"I had to be the strong one"	"My needs don't matter"	Ignoring pain, delaying care, burnout

Trauma is not defined by the **event itself,** but by the **meanings** the mind and body had to create in order to survive.

CLINICAL LENS: ASKING A DIFFERENT QUESTION

When a mother presents with distress around feeding, we can ask:

Not: What is wrong with her?
But: What has she lived through, and how has her body learned to adapt?

This shift in question is central to trauma-informed breastfeeding medicine.

CLINICAL REFLECTION: ACES AND THE INVISIBLE LOAD

ACE research does not give clinicians a script – it offers a lens. It helps explain why some parents struggle to bond, why a carefully supported birth may still feel terrifying, and why breastfeeding can trigger unexpected distress.

The goal is not to diagnose ACEs, but to deepen clinical curiosity and compassion. Asking "What happened to you?" – even silently, in our own reasoning – can shift encounters away from judgment and toward understanding.

Our role is not to treat ACEs themselves, but to recognise their echoes, to create relational safety, and to walk gently with parents whose nervous systems are still recovering from stories that began long before pregnancy. Increasingly, perinatal mental health literature emphasises that this recognition is a shared responsibility across disciplines, rather than the sole domain of specialist services.[16-18]

REFERENCES

3 Felitti VJ, Anda RF, Nordenberg D, Williamson DF, Spitz AM, Edwards V, et al. Relationship of childhood abuse and household dysfunction to many of the leading causes of death in adults. The Adverse Childhood Experiences (ACE) Study. Am J Prev Med. 1998;14(4):245–58.

4 Kolk vd. The body keeps the score: brain, mind, and body in the healing of trauma. New York: Viking; 2014.

8 Kendall-Tackett K, Cong Z, Hale TW. Depression, sleep quality, and maternal well-being in postpartum women with a history of sexual assault: a comparison of breastfeeding, mixed-feeding, and formula-feeding mothers. Breastfeed Med. 2013;8(1):16–22.

9 Miller ES, Fleming O, Ekpe EE, Grobman WA, Heard-Garris N. Association Between Adverse Childhood Experiences and Adverse Pregnancy Outcomes. Obstet Gynecol. 2021;138(5):770–6.

10 Mamun A, Biswas T, Scott J, Sly PD, McIntyre HD, Thorpe K, et al. Adverse childhood experiences, the risk of pregnancy complications and adverse pregnancy outcomes: a systematic review and meta-analysis. BMJ Open. 2023;13(8):e063826.

11 Swedo EA, D'Angelo DV, Fasula AM, Clayton HB, Ports KA. Associations of Adverse Childhood Experiences With Pregnancy and Infant Health. Am J Prev Med. 2023;64(4):512–24.

12 Roubinov DS, Luecken LJ, Curci SG, Somers JA, Winstone LK. A prenatal programming perspective on the intergenerational transmission of maternal adverse childhood experiences to offspring health problems. Am Psychol. 2021;76(2):337–49.

13 Racine N, Plamondon A, Madigan S, McDonald S, Tough S. Maternal Adverse Childhood Experiences and Infant Development. Pediatrics. 2018;141(4).

14 Johnson S, Kasparian NA, Cullum AS, Flanagan T, Ponting C, Kowalewski L, et al. Addressing Adverse Childhood and Adult Experiences During Prenatal Care. Obstet Gynecol. 2023;141(6):1072–87.

15 Borg LE, Alhusen JL. A Review of Factors that Serve to Protect Pregnant and Post-partum Women from Negative Outcomes Associated with Adverse Childhood Experiences. Matern Child Health J. 2023;27(9):1503–17.

16 Isobel S. Trauma and the perinatal period: A review of the theory and practice of trauma-sensitive interactions for nurses and midwives. Nurs Open. 2023;10(12):7585–95.

17 Sperlich M, Seng JS, Li Y, Taylor J, Bradbury-Jones C. Integrating Trauma-Informed Care Into Maternity Care Practice: Conceptual and Practical Issues. J Midwifery Womens Health. 2017;62(6):661–72.

18 Kezelman C, Stavropoulos P. Practice guidelines for treatment of complex trauma and trauma-informed care. Sydney: Blue Knot Foundation; 2012.

CHAPTER 3:

Infant Feeding in the Context of Trauma

"There is no such thing as a baby.

There is a baby and someone."

~ Dr Donald Winnicott

THE INTERSECTION OF TRAUMA AND BREASTFEEDING

Breastfeeding is a profoundly intimate act – rich in symbolism, cultural expectations, and physiological significance. For those who have experienced trauma, particularly developmental trauma or childhood sexual abuse (CSA), this intimacy can feel fraught or even unbearable. The expectation to "nourish perfectly" often collides with longstanding feelings of unworthiness, fear of exposure, and loss of bodily autonomy. For many survivors, infant feeding becomes not only a practical task but a psychological battleground.[2, 4, 20, 21]

Breastfeeding requires trust – in one's body, in the process, and in those offering care. It requires flexibility, surrender, and an ability to tolerate unpredictability. Yet trauma survivors may have learned from a young age that their body is not safe, that touch is dangerous, and that control is essential for survival. These internalised patterns can be challenged – sometimes painfully – by the act of feeding a baby.[2, 4]

THE EVIDENCE BASE: TRAUMA AND BREASTFEEDING OUTCOMES

While this complexity has long been described in qualitative literature, more recent evidence confirms a consistent association between traumatic experiences and breastfeeding outcomes. A 2025 systematic review examining traumatic childbirth and birth-related post-traumatic stress disorder found a clear negative relationship with breastfeeding initiation, duration, and maternal self-efficacy.[22] These findings reinforce that breastfeeding difficulties following trauma are not a matter of motivation or intention, but of neurobiological, psychological, and relational safety.

Importantly, this association does not imply inevitability. Rather, it highlights the mediating role of care. When breastfeeding is supported within trauma-informed, respectful, and emotionally safe environments, the negative impact of trauma may be buffered. In this context, breastfeeding becomes not a test of resilience, but a relational process shaped by the presence or absence of safety.[22-24]

Studies have demonstrated that both maternal lifetime PTSD and birth-related traumatisation are associated with numerous adverse maternal and infant outcomes, including pregnancy-related anxieties, traumatic birth experience, anxiety and depressive disorders after delivery, and in cases of interpersonal trauma, infant feeding disorders. Women with birth-related traumatisation and postpartum depression show additional associations with infant feeding and sleeping problems.[20]

NEUROBIOLOGICAL MECHANISMS: HOW TRAUMA AFFECTS LACTATION

Trauma affects far more than memory and emotion. It influences neurobiology, hormonal regulation, stress physiology, attachment systems, and bodily responses to touch and intimacy. This is highly relevant in the context of breastfeeding, which is itself a deeply neurobiological and relational process.

The Oxytocin System and Trauma

Oxytocin plays a central role in lactation, maternal behaviour, bonding, and stress regulation. During breastfeeding, oxytocin is released in pulsatile bursts, particularly in the early postpartum period, before gradually shifting into a more sustained pattern as lactation becomes established.[25] Oxytocin release is essential for milk ejection and is associated with elevated prolactin levels, reduced cortisol and ACTH levels, enhanced sociability, and reduced anxiety.[25]

In uncomplicated circumstances, this neurohormonal response promotes relaxation, emotional connection, and maternal responsiveness. Breastfeeding therefore involves not only nutrition, but also regulation of the maternal stress response system.

However, trauma exposure and PTSD can alter the functioning of the oxytocinergic system. [26] Survivors of developmental trauma or childhood sexual abuse often have nervous systems organised around hypervigilance and threat detection rather than safety and regulation. In these individuals, bodily closeness, touch, vulnerability, and dependency may feel emotionally complex or unsafe.

Peripartum neurobiological changes involving oxytocin are closely linked to maternal adaptation after birth, including bonding, emotional regulation, and lactation.[27] These same systems are also implicated in trauma processing and stress responses. As a result, breastfeeding may become a site where nurturing physiology and trauma physiology intersect.

This may help explain why breastfeeding experiences among trauma survivors are so variable. Some mothers describe feeding as calming, regulating, and healing. Others experience breastfeeding as emotionally overwhelming, dysregulating, or triggering. For many, both experiences coexist simultaneously.

Animal studies have demonstrated that peripartum stress can impair maternal postpartum behaviours and bonding responses, while activation of the oxytocinergic system in the early postpartum period may partially buffer or reverse some of these effects.[27] Human studies similarly suggest that oxytocin may have restorative neurobiological and psychological effects, including improved maternal-infant bonding and reductions in some PTSD symptoms.[27, 28]

At the same time, the relationship between oxytocin and trauma is not straightforward. Some studies have demonstrated that intranasal oxytocin administration may increase fear processing or worsen mood symptoms in women with acute trauma exposure or postpartum depression.[27] These findings suggest that oxytocin's effects are highly context-dependent and influenced by factors such as acute distress, prior trauma exposure, intrapartum experiences, and attachment history.[27, 29]

Clinically, this complexity is important to recognise. Breastfeeding is often culturally framed as instinctive, calming, and universally rewarding. For trauma survivors, however, the physiological and emotional intensity of feeding may activate competing neurobiological responses — connection and threat, nurturing and hypervigilance, closeness and fear.

Difficulties relaxing into breastfeeding should therefore not be interpreted as resistance, failure, or lack of maternal attachment. In many cases, these responses reflect a nervous system attempting to reconcile caregiving with prior experiences of danger or loss of bodily autonomy.

At the same time, with adequate safety, support, and relational care, breastfeeding may also provide opportunities for regulation, reconnection, and healing. The same neurobiological systems involved in trauma responses may, under supportive conditions, contribute to repair and attachment.

The Stress Response: Cortisol and Lactation

Maternal stress and elevated cortisol levels can significantly impair lactation through multiple mechanisms. Acute physical and mental stress can impair the milk ejection reflex by reducing the release of oxytocin during a feed.[30] If this occurs repeatedly, it could reduce milk production by preventing full emptying of the breast at each feed.[30]

Maternal and foetal stress during labour and delivery, such as urgent caesarean sections or long duration of labour in vaginal deliveries, are associated with delayed onset of lactation.[30, 31] The prolonged duration of birth causes fatigue in both mother and infant, leading to late start of lactation and reduction in breastfeeding frequency.[31] Stress increases cortisol levels and negatively affects milk production, which adversely affects breastfeeding success and lactogenesis.[31]

Interestingly, breastfeeding itself has stress-buffering effects. Both nursing and mechanical expression of breastmilk are associated with equivalent declines in maternal cortisol concentration, indicating an effect of milk letdown on circulating cortisol independent of infant contact.[23] Self-reported maternal stress is associated with higher pre-session cortisol concentrations, as well as with a larger drop in cortisol following nursing or pumping.[23]

However, maternal psychological stress affects the relationship between cortisol and prolactin in human milk. A positive association exists between salivary and milk cortisol, while a negative relationship is observed between salivary cortisol and milk prolactin.[32] This suggests that maternal psychological stress may affect hormones transported via milk that can program infant development in the early postnatal period.[32]

Trauma exposure is associated with dysregulation of the body's stress responses. Increased prenatal depressive symptoms are related to elevated prenatal cortisol awakening response and moderate the relationship between interpersonal trauma exposure and greater prenatal cortisol awakening response.[33] A significant negative correlation exists between prenatal depressive symptoms and breastfeeding frequency, suggesting that women at risk for breastfeeding difficulty may be identified prenatally.[33]

COMMON THEMES IN INFANT FEEDING AFTER ABUSE

Qualitative studies exploring infant feeding experiences of women with histories of childhood sexual abuse provide rich insight into lived experience. Though small in sample size, these studies reveal consistent and profound themes.[34]

Shame

Across qualitative accounts, shame emerges as a dominant and persistent experience. Women describe shame related to their bodies, their breastfeeding experiences, and their perceived failures as mothers. This shame is not only a legacy of abuse, but is often compounded when breastfeeding does not unfold as hoped.[30, 34]

"I was so ashamed of my body. Here I am, a failure again."[34]

For many, difficulty breastfeeding reinforced deeply entrenched beliefs of inadequacy and self-blame. This shame can be particularly intense given societal and cultural pressures around "successful" breastfeeding and the medicalisation of infant feeding practices.

Touch

Touch, in any form, may be overwhelming or triggering for survivors of childhood trauma and sexual abuse. [30, 34]

- Self-touch:

Women often avoided touching their own bodies, particularly areas associated with abuse.

"Because of the negative body image, I was never comfortable with touching my body at different places."[34]

- Infant touch:

The constant physical contact required in early parenting, especially breastfeeding, could become intolerable.

"I was touched-out... I'd had all the physical contact I could possibly take in those six weeks."[34]

- Medical touch:

Routine clinical procedures were sometimes experienced as violations when consent or explanation was lacking.

"I didn't expect some of the intrusive touching in the hospital. That was really traumatising for me. The nudity... I hadn't anticipated that."[34]

Trauma-informed care recognises that parents have reported a range of experiences during pregnancy and the transition to parenting that are reminiscent of the original trauma and consequently "trigger" trauma responses, including sounds (e.g., door closing, women calling out in labor), particular smells (e.g., coffee, urine), visual cues (e.g., KY jelly), sensory experiences (e.g., abdominal and vaginal examinations, breastfeeding), or restraint.[35] These experiences can be intensified if the parent has limited control or choice, the carer is perceived as "insensitive" or "uncaring," or a combination of these.[35]

Breasts and Body Image

The relationship women had with their breasts was often shaped by abuse history. Breasts were frequently associated with the abuse itself, and using them to feed an infant could feel confronting or unsafe.[34] For some women, breasts were viewed as functional objects disconnected from their sense of self, while for others, the sexualisation of breasts during abuse made breastfeeding feel inherently unsafe or shameful.

Women with histories of CSA more often described complications associated with breastfeeding. Mastitis and pain were reported significantly more often by women after CSA.[36] For 20% of women after CSA, breastfeeding was a trigger for memories of CSA.[36]

Dissociation

Dissociation emerged as a common coping mechanism. For some women, it was the only way breastfeeding could continue. Dissociation – in which awareness narrows, sensation blunts, and the body prepares for threat – is a well-described survival response when physical escape is not possible.[4, 20, 36]

"I didn't really have a body. I was a head with legs... the breasts were functional for that time."[34]

While dissociation enabled continued feeding, it came at significant cost. Breastfeeding became a disembodied act - performed but not felt - disrupting connection to both self and baby. Fifty-eight percent of women with CSA reported dissociation when breastfeeding, highlighting the prevalence of this coping mechanism.[36]

Medical Mistrust

Childhood abuse represents a profound betrayal by someone in a position of power. This often translates into medical mistrust in adulthood. Vulnerability during pregnancy, birth, and breastfeeding - particularly during intimate or exposed procedures - may feel unsafe. Even benign touch, if unannounced or non-consensual, can evoke fear or dissociation.[2, 21, 34]

This mistrust can manifest as difficulty accepting help from healthcare providers, reluctance to disclose difficulties with breastfeeding, or avoidance of medical care altogether. The power differential inherent in the patient-provider relationship may mirror dynamics from the original abuse, making it difficult for survivors to advocate for themselves or set boundaries.

THE POSSIBILITY OF HEALING

Trauma does not preclude healing. In Wood and Van Esterik's study, some women described their birth and breastfeeding experiences as transformative.

"This is what my body was designed for."[34]

Through breastfeeding, they were able to reclaim their bodies as sources of nourishment and strength, rather than harm. This duality - breastfeeding as both distressing and reparative – is central to understanding trauma-informed infant feeding care.[21, 34] Patients with a history of sexual trauma may choose not to breastfeed, but those who do often report positive bodily connections while breastfeeding and feelings of empowerment by their choice to do so.[37] This highlights the importance of supporting informed choice and autonomy in infant feeding decisions.

CSA, ACES, AND BREASTFEEDING PATTERNS: WHAT THE RESEARCH SHOWS

A growing body of quantitative research has examined how CSA and broader adverse childhood experiences influence breastfeeding intentions, initiation, and duration. While findings are sometimes mixed, consistent patterns emerge.

Women with histories of CSA or high ACE scores are more likely to:

- Intend to breastfeed
- Initiate breastfeeding
- Discontinue breastfeeding earlier

This paradox may reflect a strong desire to "get it right" as a parent, alongside internal and external barriers that make sustained breastfeeding difficult.[8, 36, 38-43]

Recent synthesis research suggests that traumatic childbirth and trauma-related post-traumatic stress symptoms may further compound these challenges by undermining maternal confidence, disrupting oxytocin-mediated processes, and amplifying stress responses during feeding.[22]

The intergenerational cycle of violence demonstrates detrimental and prolonged effects that traverse childhood to motherhood. Women who experienced either childhood abuse or prenatal intimate partner violence were more likely to experience negative emotional childbirth memories.[44] Not continuing to exclusively breastfeed at three months postpartum was strongly associated with prenatal depression, young age, and perceived low social status during pregnancy.[37]

Importantly, perceived strong connectedness among extended family members and social networks (i.e., nexus among family, friends, and neighbourhood) provided a buffering effect by preventing exclusive breastfeeding termination.[44] This highlights the protective role of social connectedness in improving breastfeeding practice.

HOW DEVELOPMENTAL TRAUMA SHAPES BREASTFEEDING DYNAMICS

Mothers with complex trauma histories may approach parenting with an intense need to do everything "right." This can manifest as:[45]

- Hyper-control over feeding schedules or routines – rigid adherence to feeding times, difficulty responding to flexibility to infant cues
- Difficulty tolerating unpredictability or deviation from plan – distress when feeding doesn't go as expected
- Discomfort with mess, chaos, or bodily fluids – heightened disgust responses or need for cleanliness
- Difficulty setting boundaries – either hyper-vigilant or over-accommodating in response to infant needs
- A persistent sense of being inherently different or broken – feeling fundamentally flawed as a mother
- Heightened sensitivity to perceived failure or criticism – interpreting normal or common breastfeeding challenges as personal inadequacy

Breastfeeding challenges many of these adaptations. It requires surrender. It invites touch. It is unpredictable and embodied. For trauma survivors, this combination can feel overwhelming or intolerable.[2, 4]

CLINICAL IMPLICATIONS: TRAUMA-INFORMED BREASTFEEDING SUPPORT

As clinicians, we cannot change a person's past – but we can profoundly influence how safe they feel in the present. Trauma-informed care asks us to assume the possibility of trauma and adjust our approach accordingly.[2, 45, 46]

Understanding Trauma-Informed Care

Trauma-informed care is a whole system strategy that: realizes the impact of trauma; recognises the signs and symptoms; responds through integrating trauma knowledge into policies, procedures, and practices; and resists traumatisation through skills training and best-practice approaches.[35] It seeks to increase awareness of trauma responses and where possible reduce practices that may exacerbate or trigger trauma responses.

Practical Principles

1. Emphasise Consent and Autonomy

- Always ask before touching
- Explain each step before performing any examination or procedure
- Offer genuine choices and respect decisions
- Recognise that declining breastfeeding or choosing to stop may be a protective decision

2. Be Attuned to Shame

- Use affirming, non-corrective language
- Validate effort, not just outcome
- Avoid comparison with other mothers or idealised breastfeeding experiences
- Normalise challenges and difficulties

3. Respect Boundaries

- Let the parent lead interactions
- Do not pressure continuation if feeding is emotionally damaging
- Acknowledge that stopping may be protective, not a failure
- Recognise signs of distress or dissociation and respond with sensitivity

4. Screen Gently

- Use universal, non-intrusive questions
- Never push for disclosure
- Respect when survivors do not wish or are unable to discuss their experiences
- Focus on resilience rather than pathology

5. Create a Sense of Safety

- Calm tone, predictable movements, grounded presence
- Minimize unexpected touch or procedures
- Provide privacy and control over the environment
- Avoid restraint (physical or pharmacological) when possible

6. Support the Whole Feeding Journey

- Offer compassionate guidance for mixed or formula feeding
- Reassure parents that attachment is not defined by milk alone
- Recognise that positive support, such as encouragement and advice from healthcare staff, is beneficial after birth trauma, enabling mothers to heal and recover from their experiences and supporting bonding with their infant[47]
- Understand that negative experiences, such as pressure from healthcare staff or challenges when breastfeeding, have a detrimental perceived impact on mental health outcomes, leading mothers to seek further breastfeeding and wellbeing support following a traumatic birth[47]

CONCLUSION: HOLDING BOTH TRUTHS

For many survivors, breastfeeding is one of the hardest things they will ever do. And for some, it becomes a gateway to healing. Both truths can coexist. As providers, our task is not to push or to fix. It is to witness, to honour, and to walk alongside. To help our patients feel not only competent, but safe. And to hold space for their stories - even the ones they do not yet have words for.

The principles of trauma-informed care should be used when counselling about breastfeeding. By creating environments of safety, respect, and genuine choice, we can support all parents in their infant feeding journey — whether that involves breastfeeding, formula feeding, or a combination of both. The goal is not perfect breastfeeding, but rather supporting the parent-infant relationship in whatever form nourishment takes.

REFERENCES

2 Kimberg L, Wheeler M. Trauma and Trauma-Informed Care. 2019. p. 25–56.

4 Kolk vd. The body keeps the score: brain, mind, and body in the healing of trauma. New York: Viking; 2014.

8 Kendall-Tackett K, Cong Z, Hale TW. Depression, sleep quality, and maternal well-being in postpartum women with a history of sexual assault: a comparison of breastfeeding, mixed-feeding, and formula-feeding mothers. Breastfeed Med. 2013;8(1):16–22.

19 Purkiewicz A, Regin KJ, Pietrzak-Fiećko R. Breastfeeding in the Context of Trauma and Previous Psychological Experiences: A Narrative Review. Nutrients. 2026;18(3).

20 Martini J, Asselmann E, Weidner K, Knappe S, Rosendahl J, Garthus-Niegel S. Prospective Associations of Lifetime Post-traumatic Stress Disorder and Birth-Related Traumatization With Maternal and Infant Outcomes. Front Psychiatry. 2022;13:842410.

21 Channell Doig A, Jasczynski M, Fleishman JL, Aparicio EM. Breastfeeding Among Mothers Who Have Experienced Childhood Maltreatment: A Review. J Hum Lact. 2020;36(4):710–22.

22 Cavallé-Abasolo E, Dikmen-Yildiz P, Gómez-Gómez I, Barros-Martins L, Motrico E. Impact of Traumatic Childbirth and Birth-Related Posttraumatic Stress Disorder on Breastfeeding Outcomes: A Systematic Review of Longitudinal and Cohort Studies. Birth. 2025;52(4):553–71.

23 Beery AK, Jackson B, Halstead E, Windorski SM, Nnodim-Amadi C, Upin E. Acute decrease in mothers' cortisol following nursing and milk expression. Horm Behav. 2023;153:105387.

24 Wheeler A, Sweeting F, Mayers A, Brown A, Farrington S. Improving perinatal mental health outcomes: The role of support in assisting breastfeeding experiences following birth trauma. Midwifery. 2026;152:104668.

25 Uvnäs Moberg K, Ekström-Bergström A, Buckley S, Massarotti C, Pajalic Z, Luegmair K, et al. Maternal plasma levels of oxytocin during breastfeeding-A systematic review. PLoS One. 2020;15(8):e0235806.

26 Engel S, Klusmann H, Laufer S, Pfeifer AC, Ditzen B, van Zuiden M, et al. Trauma exposure, posttraumatic stress disorder and oxytocin: A meta-analytic investigation of endogenous concentrations and receptor genotype. Neurosci Biobehav Rev. 2019;107:560–601.

27 Witteveen AB, Stramrood CAI, Henrichs J, Flanagan JC, van Pampus MG, Olff M. The oxytocinergic system in PTSD following traumatic childbirth: endogenous and exogenous oxytocin in the peripartum period. Arch Womens Ment Health. 2020;23(3):317–29.

28 Sharma SR, Gonda X, Dome P, Tarazi FI. What's Love Got to do with it: Role of oxytocin in trauma, attachment and resilience. Pharmacol Ther. 2020;214:107602.

29 Donadon MF, Martin-Santos R, Osório FL. The Associations Between Oxytocin and Trauma in Humans: A Systematic Review. Front Pharmacol. 2018;9:154.

30 Dewey KG. Maternal and fetal stress are associated with impaired lactogenesis in humans. J Nutr. 2001;131(11):3012s–5s.

31 Karakoyunlu Ö, Ejder Apay S, Gürol A. The effect of pain, stress, and cortisol during labor on breastfeeding success. Dev Psychobiol. 2019;61(7):979–87.

32 Matyas M, Apanasewicz A, Krzystek-Korpacka M, Jamrozik N, Cierniak A, Babiszewska-Aksamit M, et al. The association between maternal stress and human milk concentrations of cortisol and prolactin. Sci Rep. 2024;14(1):28115.

33 Bengtson L, Aubuchon-Endsley NL. Prenatal depression moderates the relationship between maternal trauma exposure and cortisol production and predicts breastfeeding behavior. Women Health. 2023;63(5):334–45.

34 Wood K, Van Esterik P. Infant feeding experiences of women who were sexually abused in childhood. Can Fam Physician. 2010;56(4):e136–41.

35 Jones KA, Freijah I, Brennan SE, McKenzie JE, Bright TM, Fiolet R, et al. Interventions from pregnancy to two years after birth for parents experiencing complex post-traumatic stress disorder and/or with childhood experience of maltreatment. Cochrane Database Syst Rev. 2023;5(5):Cd014874.

36 Elfgen C, Hagenbuch N, Görres G, Block E, Leeners B. Breastfeeding in Women Having Experienced Childhood Sexual Abuse. J Hum Lact. 2017;33(1):119–27.

37 Caring for Patients Who Have Experienced Trauma: ACOG Committee Opinion, Number 825. Obstetrics & Gynecology. 2021;137(4):e94–e9.

38 Prentice JC, Lu MC, Lange L, Halfon N. The association between reported childhood sexual abuse and breastfeeding initiation. J Hum Lact. 2002;18(3):219–26.

39 Sørbø MF, Lukasse M, Brantsæter AL, Grimstad H. Past and recent abuse is associated with early cessation of breast feeding: results from a large prospective cohort in Norway. BMJ Open. 2015;5(12):e009240.

40 Coles J, Anderson A, Loxton D. Breastfeeding Duration after Childhood Sexual Abuse: An Australian Cohort Study. J Hum Lact. 2016;32(3):Np28–35.

41 Ukah UV, Adu PA, De Silva DA, von Dadelszen P. The Impact of a History of Adverse Childhood Experiences on Breastfeeding Initiation and Exclusivity: Findings from a National Population Health Survey. Breastfeed Med. 2016;11:544–50.

42 McCloskey RJ, Pei F. Associations Between Mothers' Adverse Childhood Experiences, Material Hardship, and Breastfeeding Challenges in the United States. J Hum Lact. 2022;38(4):651–60.

43 Watson C, Wei J, Varnado N, Rios N, Flanagan T, Alabaster A, et al. Adverse Childhood Experiences and Early and Continued Breastfeeding: Findings from an Integrated Health Care Delivery System. J Womens Health (Larchmt). 2021;30(3):367–76.

44 Do HP, Vo TV, Murray L, Baker PRA, Murray A, Valdebenito S, et al. The influence of childhood abuse and prenatal intimate partner violence on childbirth experiences and breastfeeding outcomes. Child Abuse Negl. 2022;131:105743.

45 Barriers to Breastfeeding: Supporting Initiation and Continuation of Breastfeeding: ACOG Committee Opinion, Number 821. Obstetrics & Gynecology. 2021;137(2):e54–e62.

46 Forkey H, Szilagyi M, Kelly ET, Duffee J. Trauma-Informed Care. Pediatrics. 2021;148(2).

47 Wheeler A, Sweeting F, Mayers A, Brown A, Farrington S. The Positive Cycle of Breastfeeding-Mental Health Outcomes of Breastfeeding Mothers Following Birth Trauma. Healthcare (Basel). 2025;13(6).

CHAPTER 4:

Birth Trauma – When Expectations Shatter

"The memory of a traumatic birth can cast a long shadow over the transition to motherhood."

~ Cheryl Tatano Beck

THE DUAL NATURE OF BIRTH TRAUMA

Birth is widely celebrated as a joyful and transformative experience. Yet for many women, the reality diverges sharply from this idealised narrative. The very moment that is meant to be empowering can instead become a site of psychological harm. Birth trauma is not defined by a particular medical outcome – it is shaped by the individual's emotional experience. Trauma in the perinatal context often arises not from medical complications alone, but from a rupture between expectation and experience, control and helplessness, care and coercion.[48]

While physical trauma may be documented in medical records, psychological trauma is often held silently – in the body, memory, and evolving maternal identity. For those with a history of trauma, particularly childhood adversity, the birth process may echo earlier experiences of powerlessness or violation, leading to deep emotional distress even in the absence of physical injury.[49, 50]

As clinicians, it is essential to recognise that birth trauma is not rare. It is not confined to high-risk deliveries, nor does it affect only those with prior mental health diagnoses. Trauma may arise from loss of control, lack of consent, disrespectful care, or the shattering of deeply held expectations.[48]

WHAT IS PSYCHOLOGICAL BIRTH TRAUMA?

Psychological birth trauma refers to a birthing experience that leaves a lasting emotional imprint. While some traumatic births involve physical injury, psychological trauma may occur even when labour and delivery are clinically uncomplicated. What determines trauma is the subjective experience – how the birthing person felt, perceived, and interpreted events in the moment.[49]

This disconnect between expectation and reality may give rise to intense emotional responses such as fear, shock, helplessness, guilt, or shame. Birth trauma commonly stems from:

- Feeling stripped of control or autonomy
- Undergoing procedures without (perceived) informed consent
- Violation of personal boundaries
- Lack of emotional or physical support
- Perceived or actual threat to the life of the baby or parent
- Witnessing complications or distress without adequate explanation

Even when interventions are medically necessary, the manner in which care is communicated, consented to, and delivered profoundly shapes whether birth is later remembered as traumatic.[48, 49]

Recent integrative research has highlighted that harmful experiences during birth are often system-mediated rather than event-specific. Women describe re-traumatisation arising not only from emergencies, but from routine practices delivered without attunement, explanation, or relational safety.[51] These findings challenge clinicians to examine not only what care is provided, but how it is provided.

PREVALENCE AND RISK FACTORS

Birth trauma is more common than many assume.

- Around one in three women describe their birth as traumatic.[48]
- Between 10–44% report some degree of psychological trauma following birth.[52]
- Approximately 3.1–4% meet diagnostic criteria for childbirth-related PTSD (CB-PTSD).[53, 54]
- Subclinical CB-PTSD symptoms may affect up to 16.8% of women.[49]

In Australia, PTSD is one of the most prevalent mental health conditions in women of reproductive age, underscoring the relevance of trauma-informed perinatal care.[55]

Risk factors for birth trauma include:

- Previous trauma, including childhood sexual abuse, interpersonal violence, or medical trauma
- Complicated pregnancy or delivery
- Emergency or unplanned interventions
- Perceived or actual lack of choice or control
- Unmanaged pain or fear during labour
- Lack of partner or staff support
- Negative or unrealistic expectations of birth
- Disrespectful or non-consensual care
- Pre-existing mental health challenges

Cultural narratives that idealise birth or promote the notion of a "perfect" experience may compound distress when reality does not align with expectations. Importantly, not everyone exposed to these risk factors will experience trauma. Individual thresholds differ, and every experience deserves validation.[48, 49]

WHEN TRAUMA COMES BEFORE THE BIRTH

Women with prior trauma histories - particularly childhood abuse - are at significantly higher risk of experiencing birth as traumatic.[50] Their bodies may already carry implicit memories of threat, betrayal, or loss of control. The vulnerability inherent in labour - bodily exposure, inescapability, pain, and reliance on others - may reactivate these memories in powerful and unexpected ways.[49]

Once a nervous system has been primed by trauma, it may more readily interpret situations as dangerous, even in the absence of objective threat. Language used by healthcare providers, repeated examinations, or unanticipated touch may precipitate flashbacks, panic, or dissociation.[49]

Rates of PTSD during pregnancy and the postpartum period rise sharply with trauma exposure:

- 4.1% among women with no abuse history
- 11.4% with adult abuse
- 16.0% with childhood abuse
- 39.0% with both adult and childhood abuse histories[50]

In these contexts, birth trauma is rarely an isolated event. It often forms part of a broader picture of complex PTSD, accompanied by depression, anxiety, panic, and intrusive thoughts, all of which may complicate early parenting.[50]

Past trauma may:

- Heighten sensitivity to pain or loss of control
- Precipitate dissociation or flashbacks during labour
- Undermine perceptions of safety
- Erode trust in healthcare professionals
- Intensify self-blame when birth does not unfold as planned

One mother described her experience:

> *"The birth itself placed me into deep, deep shock... I wish somebody had told me – that as a survivor of sexual abuse, I might get thrown back into the darkness again."*

BIRTH TRAUMA AND BREASTFEEDING

Birth trauma has well-documented implications for postpartum feeding. Trauma exposure may:

- Delay or inhibit lactogenesis II
- Reduce breastfeeding duration or exclusivity
- Suppress oxytocin and prolactin release
- Impair bonding and emotional connection

- Lower maternal confidence
- Elevate cortisol levels in both mother and infant[56, 57]

Mothers with traumatic birth experiences report higher rates of feeding difficulties, earlier cessation, and emotional distress related to infant feeding.[3] Positive birth experiences, by contrast, are associated with longer breastfeeding duration and more positive feeding relationships.[57]

Recent qualitative research highlights the protective role of supportive healthcare relationships following traumatic birth. Women who felt heard, respected, and supported by healthcare staff described greater capacity to process their birth experience and engage in nurturing relationships with their infants, including through feeding.[24] Supportive care acted as a mediator of healing, even when birth itself was traumatic.

One mother reflected:

> *"After a traumatic birth, it felt like I had lost the very essence of what my body was meant to do – nourish and bond with my baby."*

Another described feeding as reparative:

> *"I really wanted to stop breastfeeding – or not even start – but the support I received in those first weeks was so healing. It helped me trust my body again."*

For the birthing parent, trauma may manifest as difficulty holding or positioning the baby, discomfort with bodily exposure during feeding, heightened anxiety about infant wellbeing, and diminished confidence in maternal identity. For the infant, dysregulation in the parent may contribute to feeding difficulties, unsettled behaviour, and heightened stress within the dyad.[56, 57]

A BROADER VIEW: ACE SCORES AND BIRTH OUTCOMES

Research demonstrates a dose-response relationship between adverse childhood experiences and adverse birth outcomes. In a cohort of 1 848 low-income women, 84.4% reported at least one ACE, and 68.2% reported multiple ACEs. Emotional neglect and childhood sexual abuse were most strongly associated with adverse outcomes.[58]

Each additional ACE was associated with:

- A 12% increase in pregnancy loss
- A 7% increase in preterm birth
- An 8% increase in low birth weight[58]

Meta-analyses have similarly identified increased risks of preterm delivery and low birth weight among women with histories of childhood maltreatment.[10, 59, 60] Seng and colleagues further demonstrated that PTSD related to childhood trauma is a stronger predictor of adverse birth outcomes than sociodemographic risk factors alone. Women with PTSD had a fourfold increase in spontaneous preterm birth, and trauma-related dissociation was independently associated with lower birth weight.[61]

CLINICAL REFLECTION: LANGUAGE, CONSENT, AND COMPASSION

As one mother reflected:

> *"I'm not happy with how it went, but I felt in control every step of the way... I'm at peace with that."*

This highlights a crucial truth: trauma is mitigated when individuals feel respected, informed, and involved in decision-making, even when outcomes are difficult.[48]

Emerging literature on re-traumatisation within perinatal services emphasises that preventable harm often arises from communication failures, power imbalances, and procedural rigidity, rather than from emergencies themselves.[15]

Clinicians can reduce harm by:

- Asking permission before touch or examination
- Explaining procedures clearly
- Offering genuine choices
- Validating distress
- Supporting flexible feeding goals

We cannot always prevent trauma, but we can minimise it. And when trauma has already occurred, sensitive, respectful care can support healing.

BIRTH AS RE-TRAUMATISATION OR REDEMPTION

For some, birth re-enacts old wounds. For others, it offers an opportunity to reclaim the body. Both experiences are valid.

One mother shared:

> *"By being able to breastfeed, I proved to myself that I could do something right."*

Our role as providers is not to eliminate all risk, but to centre the person, protect autonomy, and create conditions that allow healing rather than harm. Birth is not a single event – it is the beginning of a story that continues through feeding, bonding, and the emergence of a new parent.

REFERENCES

10 Mamun A, Biswas T, Scott J, Sly PD, McIntyre HD, Thorpe K, et al. Adverse childhood experiences, the risk of pregnancy complications and adverse pregnancy outcomes: a systematic review and meta-analysis. BMJ Open. 2023;13(8):e063826.

24 Wheeler A, Sweeting F, Mayers A, Brown A, Farrington S. Improving perinatal mental health outcomes: The role of support in assisting breastfeeding experiences following birth trauma. Midwifery. 2026;152:104668.

48 Australia BT. What is birth trauma? n.d. [Birth Trauma Australia]. Available from: https://birthtrauma.org.au/what-is-birth-trauma/.

49 Dekel S, Stuebe C, Dishy G. Childbirth Induced Posttraumatic Stress Syndrome: A Systematic Review of Prevalence and Risk Factors. Front Psychol. 2017;8:560.

50 Wosu AC, Gelaye B, Williams MA. History of childhood sexual abuse and risk of prenatal and postpartum depression or depressive symptoms: an epidemiologic review. Arch Womens Ment Health. 2015;18(5):659–71.

51 Gordon J, Hunter A, Callanan F, Kiely C, Grealish A. An Integrative Review Exploring Womens' Experiences of Retraumatization Within Perinatal Services. J Midwifery Womens Health. 2025;70(1):32–49.

52 Pidd D, Newton M, Wilson I, East C. Optimising maternity care for a subsequent pregnancy after a psychologically traumatic birth: A scoping review. Women Birth. 2023;36(5):e471–e80.

53 Grekin R, O'Hara MW. Prevalence and risk factors of postpartum posttraumatic stress disorder: a meta-analysis. Clin Psychol Rev. 2014;34(5):389–401.

54 Yildiz PD, Ayers S, Phillips L. The prevalence of posttraumatic stress disorder in pregnancy and after birth: A systematic review and meta-analysis. J Affect Disord. 2017;208:634–45.

55 McEvoy PM, Grove R, Slade T. Epidemiology of anxiety disorders in the Australian general population: findings of the 2007 Australian National Survey of Mental Health and Wellbeing. Aust N Z J Psychiatry. 2011;45(11):957–67.

56 Beck CT, Watson S. Impact of birth trauma on breast-feeding: a tale of two pathways. Nurs Res. 2008;57(4):228–36.

57 Davis AMB, Sclafani V. Birth Experiences, Breastfeeding, and the Mother-Child Relationship: Evidence from a Large Sample of Mothers. Can J Nurs Res. 2022;54(4):518–29.

58 Mersky JP, Lee CP. Adverse childhood experiences and poor birth outcomes in a diverse, low-income sample. BMC Pregnancy Childbirth. 2019;19(1):387.

59 Nesari M, Olson JK, Vandermeer B, Slater L, Olson DM. Does a maternal history of abuse before pregnancy affect pregnancy outcomes? A systematic review with meta-analysis. BMC Pregnancy Childbirth. 2018;18(1):404.

60 Kern A, Khoury B, Frederickson A, Langevin R. The associations between childhood maltreatment and pregnancy complications: A systematic review and meta-analysis. J Psychosom Res. 2022;160:110985.

61 Seng JS, Low LK, Sperlich M, Ronis DL, Liberzon I. Prevalence, trauma history, and risk for posttraumatic stress disorder among nulliparous women in maternity care. Obstet Gynecol. 2009;114(4):839–47.

CHAPTER 5:

Tiny Babies, Tremendous Stress: Trauma in the NICU Environment

"The most powerful protection against stress is a sense of being loved and supported."

~ Dr Bruce Perry

UNIMAGINABLE BEGINNINGS

Few parents picture their newborn arriving early or unwell, or being whisked into a neonatal intensive care unit (NICU). The image of skin-to-skin contact, immediate bonding, and a gentle feeding journey is abruptly replaced by medical machines, separation, and uncertainty. NICU admission is not just a medical event – it is a profoundly emotional one. For many parents, it is traumatic.

Mothers and fathers in NICU settings face fear for their baby's survival, physical separation, disruptions to bonding, uncertainty about the future, and an environment that can feel clinical, disempowering, and alien. The trauma of the NICU experience can linger – long after the baby is home.[62]

PSYCHOLOGICAL IMPACT OF THE NICU EXPERIENCE

The NICU is a setting filled with life-saving interventions, but it can also be a site of psychological injury for parents. Unlike a single traumatic event, the NICU exposes parents to repeated stressors – alarms, invasive procedures, prolonged uncertainty, and moments of helpless observation. Parents of babies in NICU are often exposed to distressing events in a repetitive and relentless way.

A large systematic review and meta-analysis by Malouf et al. documented high rates of mental health symptoms among NICU parents:[62]

- One month postpartum
  - Anxiety – 41.9%
  - PTSD – 39.9%
- 1–12 months postpartum
  - Anxiety – 26.3%
  - PTSD – 24.5%
- More than one year postpartum
  - PTSD – 27.1%

These rates far exceed community baseline prevalence. While symptoms may lessen over time, they often remain elevated, particularly when the NICU experience involves prolonged medical uncertainty, invasive care, or fear of loss.[62]

In addition to fear for their baby's health and survival, parents may face separation from partners and older children, unfamiliar environments, disrupted routines, and communication breakdowns with staff. These experiences can significantly impact mental health, the transition to parenthood, and the developing parent–infant relationship.[62]

Importantly, emerging qualitative work highlights that parents' psychological outcomes are strongly shaped by their relationships with healthcare staff. When communication is inconsistent, dismissive, or overly technical, distress is amplified. Conversely, continuity of care, clear explanations, and relational safety can buffer the psychological impact of the NICU experience, even in the context of significant medical complexity.[63]

THE NICU AND ITS DISRUPTION TO BONDING AND BREASTFEEDING

The NICU disrupts the hormonal, sensory, and relational processes that support early bonding and lactation. Parents are often physically separated from their baby during the critical early hours and days postpartum. The infant may be unable to suck, feed orally, or tolerate milk for extended periods.

Common challenges include:

- Delayed or disrupted milk production due to stress and limited early skin-to-skin contact
- Exclusive expressing for prolonged periods without the regulatory feedback of infant suckling
- Gastrointestinal immaturity delaying feeding advancement
- Inability to feed at the breast for medical or developmental reasons

- Trauma-related dissociation or depression in the parent, interfering with emotional connection

Maternal traumatic stress and depression may inhibit bonding and compound the difficulties of establishing lactation. Even once the infant is medically stable, feeding challenges may persist due to oral aversions, sensory sensitivities, or reliance on feeding tubes – all of which can disrupt the reciprocity and pleasure of feeding.[62, 64]

Recent research emphasises that breastfeeding trajectories in the NICU are not determined by motivation alone, but by the presence or absence of integrated psychological, relational, and lactation support. When parents feel emotionally held and practically supported, feeding outcomes and confidence improve.[24]

FEEDING OUTCOMES IN NICU INFANTS

Breastfeeding in the NICU is possible, but the barriers are substantial and frequently underestimated. A prospective study by Sokou et al. examining breastfeeding outcomes in NICU-admitted neonates found:[64]

- 78.1% received maternal milk in the early neonatal period
- 58.1% were exclusively breastfed by the end of the first month
- 36.9% remained exclusively breastfed by three months
- only 19.4% were exclusively breastfed at six months

These rates fall well below World Health Organization recommendations for exclusive breastfeeding to six months, highlighting the complex obstacles faced by families with hospitalised neonates.[65]

The authors emphasised that parents of NICU-admitted infants require integrated, multidisciplinary support – encompassing lactation, mental health, nursing, and medical care – to sustain breastfeeding over time. Without such support, even highly motivated parents may be unable to achieve their feeding goals.[64]

CLINICAL REFLECTION: CARING FOR NICU FAMILIES WITH COMPASSION

NICU parents are not only managing the technical demands of prematurity or illness – they are doing so while carrying the emotional weight of trauma. We must never assume that improvement in the baby's condition equates to recovery for the parent.

Qualitative case-based research highlights the importance of interprofessional, trauma-informed collaboration in NICU care. Parents report better psychological outcomes when care teams prioritise communication, shared decision-making, and consistent messaging across disciplines.[63] This relational continuity helps parents feel seen as central participants in their baby's care, rather than passive observers.

Practical ways clinicians can support NICU families include:

- acknowledging the trauma – validating fear, grief, and powerlessness
- supporting early milk expression – ideally within 1–3 hours postpartum when feasible
- providing trauma-informed lactation care – recognising that expressing milk may feel disembodied or emotionally charged
- facilitating contact – encouraging touch, skin-to-skin, and cue-based interaction as soon as medically appropriate
- protecting mental health – gentle screening for distress and timely referral for psychological support
- rebuilding confidence – reinforcing the parent's central role in their baby's care, even when proximity is limited

Supportive staff relationships are not a luxury in NICU care; they are therapeutic in their own right. Parents who experience empathy, consistency, and respect from healthcare professionals describe greater capacity to process trauma and engage confidently in caregiving and feeding, even after highly stressful neonatal admissions.[24]

CLOSING: GRIEF, GUILT, AND GRACE IN THE NICU

Parents in the NICU are doing the impossible. They are grieving the loss of the birth and postpartum experience they imagined, navigating uncertainty, and learning to parent in an intensely medicalised environment. Breastfeeding may become a source of healing - but it can also be a source of grief, frustration, or shame.

The trauma of NICU care does not end at discharge. It often walks with families long after they leave the hospital. Our role is to recognise it, name it, and support the parent-infant relationship not only medically, but emotionally - with tenderness, patience, and hope.

REFERENCES

24 Wheeler A, Sweeting F, Mayers A, Brown A, Farrington S. Improving perinatal mental health outcomes: The role of support in assisting breastfeeding experiences following birth trauma. Midwifery. 2026;152:104668.

62 Malouf R, Harrison S, Burton HAL, Gale C, Stein A, Franck LS, et al. Prevalence of anxiety and post-traumatic stress (PTS) among the parents of babies admitted to neonatal units: A systematic review and meta-analysis. EClinicalMedicine. 2022;43:101233.

63 Horan H, Ryu J, Stone J, Thurston L. Healing trauma with interprofessional collaboration and trauma-informed perinatal care: A qualitative case study. Birth. 2023;50(3):525–34.

64 Sokou R, Parastatidou S, Ioakeimidis G, Tavoulari EF, Makrogianni A, Isaakidou E, et al. Breastfeeding in Neonates Admitted to an NICU: 18-Month Follow-Up. Nutrients. 2022;14(18).

65 Organization WH. Infant and young child feeding. World Health Organisation; 2023.

CHAPTER 6:

When the Past Resurfaces – Identifying and Managing Triggers in the Perinatal Period

"The past affects the present even without our being aware of it."

~ Dr Francine Shapiro

UNDERSTANDING TRIGGERS

Trauma does not always announce itself with words – it often surfaces through the body, emotions, or sensations. In the perinatal period, the body becomes central: changing, exposed, touched, and examined. This makes it a uniquely vulnerable time for people with a history of trauma. Even in the absence of conscious memory, the body may respond with fear, shame, or dissociation when cues echo earlier harm.[66]

These cues, known as triggers, can disrupt presence, safety, and connection. They may arise during pregnancy, labour, birth, breastfeeding, or within the NICU environment. For some parents, a trigger is clear and specific. For others, it is vague or confusing – a sense that something is wrong without an obvious explanation.

Triggers do not need to be dramatic or explicit. They are highly individual and shaped by personal history. It is neither possible nor necessary to eliminate all triggers. Rather, trauma-informed care recognises their complexity and seeks to respond with flexibility, curiosity, and compassion.[66]

Recent integrative research has highlighted that many perinatal triggers are not inherent to medical care itself, but arise from how care is delivered. Women describe re-traumatisation occurring through routine interactions when consent is assumed, communication is rushed, or power imbalances are left unacknowledged.[51] Recognising triggers therefore requires attention not only to patient history, but to clinical culture and practice.

COMMON SENSORY, EMOTIONAL, AND SITUATIONAL TRIGGERS

Triggers are deeply personal, but certain patterns are frequently observed in perinatal care.

Sensory triggers may include the smell of antiseptics or blood, the sound of medical monitors, fluorescent lighting, or the sensation of sticky fluids such as milk, sweat, or blood.

Emotional triggers often arise from feelings of exposure during examinations, being the focus of attention, fear of judgment, or perceived scrutiny.

Situational triggers may include being alone in a closed room while waiting for a clinician, unexpected touch, crowded waiting rooms, physical restraint, or a loss of privacy.

Language itself can also act as a powerful trigger. Phrases such as "If you just relax, it won't hurt so much" may be intended to reassure, but for some survivors they echo language used in abusive or coercive contexts. Other commonly reported phrases include "Just lift your bottom," "Good girl," "Trust your body," or "You're doing fine" – particularly when the person does not feel fine.

For individuals whose bodies have previously been sites of harm, advice implying that their body *should* behave in a particular way may feel invalidating or unsafe. Many survivors describe a profound sense that their body has betrayed them, making such statements especially distressing.[67]

SPECIFIC PERINATAL TRIGGERS REPORTED BY SURVIVORS

Survivors commonly describe triggers across the perinatal continuum:

- Pregnancy: sensations of invasion or loss of bodily autonomy, described as "a foreign body inside me"
- Labour: repeated touch, being observed, lying flat, lack of control
- Birth: exposure of genitals, vaginal examinations, being cut or stitched
- Postpartum: milk leakage, skin-to-skin contact, loss of privacy, intrusive memories
- NICU: separation from the baby, medical jargon, helplessness, repeated alarms

One mother reflected on her experience:

> *"The birth itself placed me into deep, deep shock. I didn't expect there to be so many hands 'down there'. I wish somebody had prepared me for that... I wish somebody had told me – that as a survivor of sexual abuse, I might get thrown back into the darkness again."*

She later described her feeding experience:

> *"I then went on to breastfeed for three months and the whole thing made me feel sick but I couldn't put my finger on why... I felt so squishy, gross and vulnerable and felt like my job was to make everyone else happy."*

These responses are not unusual. They are understandable reactions to stimuli that echo earlier experiences of powerlessness or violation. Recognising these patterns allows clinicians to anticipate potential triggers and respond with greater sensitivity.

RECOGNISING TRIGGERS IN PRACTICE

We cannot prevent every trigger, but we can learn to recognise when someone has become activated. Common signs include:

- sudden withdrawal or dissociation
- tears, panic, or visible physical tension
- delayed responses or difficulty speaking
- hyper-compliance or emotional shutdown

When these signs are noticed, a gentle pause can be powerful. Simple statements such as *"You don't seem very comfortable right now – what can we do to help?"* help re-establish safety and restore agency.

Importantly, clinicians often report uncertainty about when and how to respond to trauma activation. An integrative review of perinatal clinicians' experiences found that many professionals recognise trauma responses, yet feel under-trained to address them safely[7] or worry about "opening something they cannot contain." This highlights the need for trauma-informed approaches that prioritise presence, pacing, and referral pathways rather than disclosure or resolution in the moment.

TOOLS FOR PATIENTS AND PROVIDERS

For clinicians

- Ask about triggers sensitively: *"Are there any parts of care that make you feel anxious or uncomfortable?"*
- Offer choice and control: *"Would you like me to explain before I start, or as I go?"*
- Before beginning any examination, remind the person that you can halt the examination at any time, with an agreed movement such as raising their hand, or just saying to stop
- Be mindful of language, tone, and positioning
- Consider trauma screening tools, such as the Antenatal Risk Questionnaire (ANRQ), as conversation starters rather than diagnostic instruments,[69] but ensure follow through if these tools are used so that patients are not left wondering what happens to the information that they have disclosed

For patients and parents

- Trigger diary: noting situations or sensations that provoke distress can help identify patterns
- Grounding techniques: slow breathing, naming objects in the room, holding a textured object
- Post-appointment reflection: "What moment today felt most overwhelming?"

Understanding what triggers a reaction is often the first step toward regaining a sense of control and safety. These strategies will be explored in more depth in later chapters.

CLOSING REFLECTIONS

Triggers are not flaws. They are learned survival responses shaped by earlier experiences. While we may not eliminate them, we can support parents in recognising, naming, and responding to them with compassion.

When clinicians attend not only to what care is delivered, but how it is delivered, we reduce the risk of retraumatisation and create opportunities for repair. In doing so, we offer agency, dignity, and the possibility of feeling safe in clinical spaces – sometimes for the first time.

REFERENCES

7 Callanan F, Bradshaw C, Tuohy T, Noonan M, Murphy S, Grealish A. An integrative review of how midwives are screening and assessing for trauma in women within perinatal services. PLoS One. 2025;20(7):e0327253.

51 Gordon J, Hunter A, Callanan F, Kiely C, Grealish A. An Integrative Review Exploring Womens' Experiences of Retraumatization Within Perinatal Services. J Midwifery Womens Health. 2025;70(1):32–49.

66 Kendall-Tackett K. Psychological Trauma and Breastfeeding: What We Know So Far. Medical Research Archives. 2022;10.

67 Moog NK, Buss C, Entringer S, Shahbaba B, Gillen DL, Hobel CJ, et al. Maternal Exposure to Childhood Trauma Is Associated During Pregnancy With Placental-Fetal Stress Physiology. Biol Psychiatry. 2016;79(10):831–9.

68 Beck CT, Watson S. Subsequent childbirth after a previous traumatic birth. Nurs Res. 2010;59(4):241–9.

69 COPE. Mental health care in the perinatal period: Australian clinical practice guideline. Melbourne: Centre of Perinatal Excellence (COPE); 2023.

CHAPTER 7:

The Healing Power of Breastfeeding – Physiology, Psychology and Mental Health Connections

"Love is not a state of perfect caring.

It is an active noun, like struggle."

~ Fred Rogers

BREASTFEEDING AS A SITE OF REPAIR

While breastfeeding is often framed primarily in terms of infant nutrition, it also carries profound physiological and psychological implications for the mother. For those with trauma histories, the act of breastfeeding can be complex - it may be triggering, healing, or both. Yet for many, with adequate support, breastfeeding becomes a powerful tool for emotional regulation, reconnection, and healing.

This chapter explores the neurobiology of breastfeeding, its impact on maternal mental health, and the ways in which it may interrupt cycles of trauma. Breastfeeding is not a cure - but it can provide survivors with a tangible opportunity to reclaim trust in their bodies, build confidence, and create new relational patterns. Crucially, these benefits are not inherent to breastfeeding alone, but are shaped by the quality of care, support, and autonomy surrounding the feeding experience.

NEUROBIOLOGICAL MECHANISMS: OXYTOCIN, CORTISOL, AND THE STRESS RESPONSE

When oxytocin is up, stress is down. And vice versa. A highly stressed mother will have difficulty breastfeeding - and giving birth.[8]

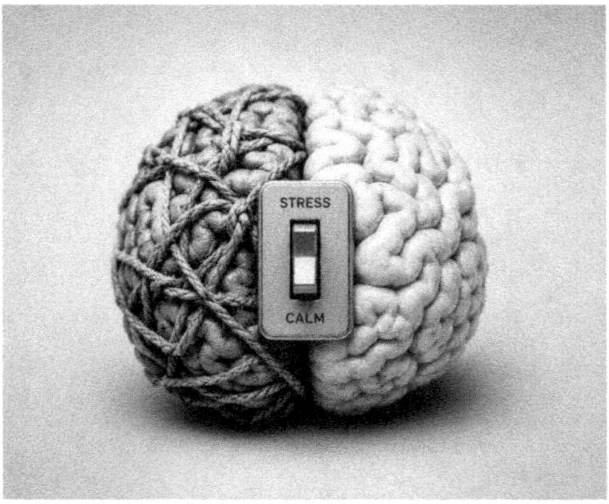

Breastfeeding activates a coordinated cascade of hormonal responses that influence both physiology and emotional state:

- Oxytocin release: Often referred to as the "love hormone," oxytocin promotes bonding, enhances maternal sensitivity, and dampens fear and anxiety responses.
- Cortisol reduction: Breastfeeding is associated with lower circulating stress hormones, supporting improved mood regulation and sleep.
- ACTH modulation: Regulation of adrenocorticotropic hormone contributes to a calmer physiological baseline.[8]

For mothers with trauma histories, these mechanisms are particularly relevant. Trauma is associated with dysregulation of the hypothalamic–pituitary–adrenal (HPA) axis and altered cortisol responses. Persistently elevated stress hormones can interfere with milk production, emotional availability, and the capacity to experience safety. Breastfeeding can help to rebalance this system when the parent feels supported, safe, and in control.

Even among women with a history of post-traumatic stress disorder, breastfeeding has been associated with lower perceived stress and improved mood compared with mixed or formula feeding.[8] Importantly, these associations are strongest when breastfeeding occurs within environments characterised by emotional safety, respectful care, and responsive support.[47]

BREASTFEEDING AND MATERNAL MENTAL HEALTH

Breastfeeding and mental health share a bidirectional relationship. Depression, anxiety, and trauma-related symptoms can interfere with breastfeeding initiation or continuation. At the same time, breastfeeding itself may actively support maternal wellbeing for some individuals:

- Improved sleep: Breastfeeding mothers often experience longer total sleep duration, despite frequent night waking.
- Reduced irritability: Exclusive breastfeeding may buffer against emotional dysregulation.

- Stabilised mood: Breastfeeding is associated with lower rates of postpartum depression.
- Increased self-efficacy: For many trauma survivors, breastfeeding can feel redemptive - a tangible experience of competence and bodily trust.

Breastfeeding does not erase trauma, but it may reduce symptom severity and function as a protective factor for emotional stability. For some survivors, it becomes one of the most empowering actions they take for their own healing.[8]

Recent qualitative research further highlights that supportive healthcare relationships play a decisive role in whether breastfeeding is experienced as burdensome or reparative. Women who felt heard, respected, and emotionally supported after birth described greater capacity to engage in breastfeeding as a healing, confidence-building experience, even following traumatic deliveries.[47]

INTERRUPTING INTERGENERATIONAL TRAUMA

Perhaps most striking is the potential for breastfeeding to interrupt the intergenerational transmission of trauma. A large longitudinal Australian cohort study involving more than 7,200 mother-infant dyads found that breastfeeding was associated with a substantially reduced risk of later child maltreatment.[70]

Mothers who breastfed for four months or longer were:

- 3.8 times less likely to neglect their children
- 2.6 times less likely to physically abuse their children

Breastfeeding strengthens maternal sensitivity and supports the development of secure attachment patterns - both powerful buffers against future trauma. While breastfeeding alone cannot protect a child from all harm, it contributes to a more responsive, attuned caregiving environment when combined with broader psychosocial support.

We often say "breast is best" in reference to infant health. This research reminds us that breastfeeding can also represent an investment in the mother's healing and the relational health of the family system.

A SURVIVOR'S STORY: BREASTFEEDING AS BOTH BURDEN AND BREAKTHROUGH

To fully appreciate the layered nature of breastfeeding after trauma, we must honour the voices of those who have lived it. For some survivors, breastfeeding becomes more than feeding – it becomes a pathway back into the body itself:

> *"To have my body used for good, to have it serve another human in the only way that a female body is meant to, was just so healing for me. Finally, my body was being used as it had been designed. After all of these years of living alongside, and at times separate to my body, I finally became one with my body once again."*

ACKNOWLEDGING COMPLEXITY

Not all trauma survivors experience breastfeeding as healing. For some, it is neutral. For others, it is deeply distressing. Healing is not linear, and there is no single right path. What matters most is choice, support, and agency.

Trauma-informed postpartum care emphasises that healing occurs not through prescribed behaviours, but through environments that prioritise safety, predictability, consent, and emotional attunement.[71] When breastfeeding is offered as an option rather than an expectation, it is more likely to become reparative rather than re-traumatising.

These stories remind us that breastfeeding is never just feeding. It may become the battleground where old wounds resurface – or the place where new narratives are written. Our role as clinicians is not to push an outcome, but to support a process. When we walk alongside our patients through grief, effort, and triumph, we help them reclaim more than feeding – we help them reclaim trust, dignity, and connection.

In the next chapter, we will explore how trauma-informed principles can be integrated across perinatal and lactation care, creating safer spaces for healing, feeding, and relationship-building.

REFERENCES

8 Kendall-Tackett K, Cong Z, Hale TW. Depression, sleep quality, and maternal well-being in postpartum women with a history of sexual assault: a comparison of breastfeeding, mixed-feeding, and formula-feeding mothers. Breastfeed Med. 2013;8(1):16–22.

47 Wheeler A, Sweeting F, Mayers A, Brown A, Farrington S. The Positive Cycle of Breastfeeding-Mental Health Outcomes of Breastfeeding Mothers Following Birth Trauma. Healthcare (Basel). 2025;13(6).

70 Strathearn L, Mamun AA, Najman JM, O'Callaghan MJ. Does breastfeeding protect against substantiated child abuse and neglect? A 15-year cohort study. Pediatrics. 2009;123(2):483–93.

71 White A, Saxer K, Raja S, Hall SL. A Trauma-informed Approach to Postpartum Care. Clin Obstet Gynecol. 2022;65(3):550–62.

CHAPTER 8:

Supporting the Breastfeeding Parent – A Trauma-Informed Approach

"Healing takes place in relationship,

but it also requires reclaiming one's

own capacity for choice."

~ Judith Herman

WHAT IS TRAUMA-INFORMED CARE?

Trauma-informed care is an approach that recognises the widespread impact of trauma and actively seeks to avoid re-traumatisation. It emphasises safety, trust, choice, collaboration, and empowerment. Rather than asking *"What is wrong with you?"*, it reframes care toward:
"What may have happened to you - and how can I help you feel safe now?"[72]

This model does not require disclosure of traumatic experiences. Instead, it creates an environment in which all patients are treated with the assumption that trauma may be present - because for many, it is. The aim is to foster healing relationships, minimise triggers, and support emotional regulation in every interaction.[72]

Importantly, trauma-informed care is not about special treatment or lowering standards of care. It is about how care is delivered - particularly in moments of vulnerability, exposure, or loss of control.

A UNIVERSAL APPROACH

"For what patients do I consider this? Everyone."

Trauma-informed care is not reserved for a select few - it is a universal approach. Given that a majority of adults report at least one adverse childhood experience, and that sexual violence is highly prevalent among women, it is statistically likely that many breastfeeding parents we support carry trauma histories.[66, 69]

Even when trauma is not disclosed, behaviours may offer clues: discomfort with touch, difficulty making eye contact, abrupt emotional responses, or vague distress.[73] In these moments, knowing the story is not essential. Responding in a way that assumes the possibility of trauma is often enough to establish safety and trust.

If a parent does disclose trauma, it is important to recognise that disclosure is rarely about telling the story. It is usually about seeking support - for themselves and for their baby. That disclosure deserves respect, containment, and care.

ASKING ABOUT TRAUMA: IF, WHEN, AND HOW

You can ask - but you are not entitled to the information. The goal is not to uncover trauma, but to provide care that acknowledges its possible presence.

If you do ask, consider the following principles:

- Use behavioural rather than diagnostic language
- Normalise the questions as part of routine care
- Be mindful of language - terms such as *"survivor"* are associated with higher response rates than *"victim"*
- Ensure that written disclosures are followed up
- Consider safety and context, particularly if a partner is present

When asking about trauma histories, questions that focus on specific experiences are often more reliable and easier for people to answer than questions that require them to identify with a label. For example, rather than asking, "Have you experienced trauma?" consider asking, "Before the age of 18, did anyone ever physically hurt, threaten, or sexually touch you in a way that made you feel unsafe?" or "Have you experienced physical assault, sexual violence, or other frightening events at any point in your life?" Behavioural questions reduce the need for individuals to decide whether their experiences "count" as trauma and may improve the accuracy of disclosure.

Screening tools such as the Antenatal Risk Questionnaire (ANRQ) may be helpful as conversation starters, not as checklists to be completed and forgotten.[69] Importantly, if you do request questionnaires to be completed, it is imperative that you follow through and address the responses.

LANGUAGE AND PHRASING SUGGESTIONS

"These are questions I ask everyone. We know many people have had past experiences that can affect birth or feeding. Is there anything you'd like me to know so I can support you better?"

"You don't seem very comfortable right now. What can I do to help?"

"Thank you for trusting me with that. Please let me know how I can help you feel more at ease."

Language is never neutral. It can soothe – or it can wound.

CREATING SAFETY THROUGH CHOICE AND CONTROL

Safety is the cornerstone of trauma-informed care. In breastfeeding support, this may involve:

- Explicit consent before touch
- Offering choice in positioning, environment, and pacing
- Supporting privacy through space, clothing, or alternatives
- Validating discomfort without pressure to "push through"

Empowerment is not about encouraging endurance. It is about restoring agency.

Research on re-traumatisation in perinatal services consistently identifies lack of consent, rushed care, and assumed compliance as key contributors to harm – even in otherwise well-intentioned systems.[7] Small shifts in practice can therefore have disproportionate protective effects.

COMPASSIONATE COMMUNICATION: HOLDING SPACE

To hold space is to remain grounded, present, and non-judgmental in the face of vulnerability. It is less about fixing and more about witnessing.

"Patients don't care how much you know until they know how much you care."

~ Theodore Roosevelt

Holding space involves:

- Active listening without rushing to solutions
- Reflecting emotional content, not just facts
- Curiosity over assumption
- Empathy over expertise

Listening is intentional. Hearing is passive. When we truly listen, we attend not only to words, but to pauses, tone, and what may be left unsaid.[74]

AVOIDING ASSUMPTIONS

Assumptions silence patients. When we fill in the gaps for them – about their needs, motivations, or capacity – we remove their voice.

Instead:

- Ask rather than presume
- Use open-ended questions
- Recognise that responses may reflect history, not resistance
- Become comfortable with silence and making space for time to respond

LANGUAGE AS A CLINICAL TOOL

Trauma-informed care asks us to pause and ask:

- *"What else am I communicating here?"*
- *"How might this be received?"*

Reactivity says: *This is about me.*
Responsiveness says: *This is about you.*

Plain, respectful language reduces power imbalance. Clarity is a form of kindness.

WHEN WORDS WOUND: A SURVIVOR'S STORY

Even with good intentions, language can cause harm. One survivor reflected:

"As she was stitching me up, she asked who the rapist was. The pity on her face was the last thing I needed. Survivors are triumphant – the last thing we need is pity."

This story reminds us that trauma-informed care is not about walking on eggshells. It is about walking with intention.

WHAT MOTHERS WITH TRAUMA WANT YOU TO KNOW

"We don't want to be defined by our experiences."

"I want you to know – but I don't want your pity."

Disclosure is rare and measured. You are not opening Pandora's box. If a disclosure arises and you feel unsure how to respond:

- *"Thank you for telling me. That's a lot to carry."*
- *"I want to support you, and sharing this helps me to understand how I can best support you."*

COMMON CONCERNS FROM CLINICIANS

- *"What if I open something I can't contain?"*
- *"I don't have time."*
- *"I feel out of my depth."*

These concerns are valid. Trauma-informed care does not require becoming a trauma therapist. It requires adjusting how care is delivered.

Containment strategies include:

- Naming time limits

- Being transparent about your own scope
- Offering follow-up or referral

SYSTEMIC BARRIERS AND SMALL SHIFTS

Trauma-informed care exists within systems that are often time-pressured and under-resourced. This is where small changes matter most:

- Asking for consent before touch
- Naming discomfort without fixing it
- Offering a few minutes of undivided presence
- Sitting rather than standing

Care does not need to be perfect to be trauma-informed. It needs to be predictable, respectful, and emotionally attuned.

CLOSING REFLECTIONS

Holding space is a clinical posture – not a technique. It is how we sit, how we listen, how we respond. It is a quiet act of advocacy that reminds parents they are safe, seen, and not alone.

Healing does not only happen through interventions. It happens in relationship – in moments where dignity is restored and agency returned.

REFERENCES

7 Callanan F, Bradshaw C, Tuohy T, Noonan M, Murphy S, Grealish A. An integrative review of how midwives are screening and assessing for trauma in women within perinatal services. PLoS One. 2025;20(7):e0327253.

66 Kendall-Tackett K. Psychological Trauma and Breastfeeding: What We Know So Far. Medical Research Archives. 2022;10.

69 COPE. Mental health care in the perinatal period: Australian clinical practice guideline. Melbourne: Centre of Perinatal Excellence (COPE); 2023.

72 SAMHSA. SAMHSA's Concept of Trauma and Guidance for a Trauma-Informed Approach. Rockville, MD; 2014. Report No.: (SMA) 14-4884.

73 Levine PA. In an Unspoken Voice: How the Body Releases Trauma and Restores Goodness. Berkeley: North Atlantic Books; 2010

74 Nichols MP, Straus MB. The Lost Art of Listening: How Learning to Listen Can Improve Relationships. 3rd ed. New York: Guilford Press; 2021.

CHAPTER 9:

From Awareness to Action - Therapeutic Interventions for Establishing Safety

"Being heard is so close to being loved that for the average person they are almost indistinguishable."

~ David Augsburger

UNDERSTANDING THE BODY AFTER TRAUMA

When someone experiences trauma, particularly repeated or early trauma, their body often becomes both a battleground and a barometer. Survivors may carry chronic muscle tension, pain, gastrointestinal symptoms, or fatigue. Their nervous systems may remain primed for danger, and their connection to bodily sensations may feel disrupted, unsafe, or unpredictable.

This is particularly important to recognise in lactation support. Breastfeeding is not just a physical act – it is an embodied experience. For mothers with trauma histories, bodily sensations such as let-down, infant touch, milk leakage, or engorgement may feel overwhelming, confusing, or distressing rather than neutral or pleasurable.

As van der Kolk famously described, *"the body keeps the score."*[75] Without involving the body in healing, many trauma survivors remain stuck, even when they intellectually understand what has happened to them. Yet for these same individuals, reconnecting with the body can feel frightening or intolerable.

Providers must approach this tension with care. Survivors may need time, privacy, and gentle guidance to tolerate being present in their bodies during feeding. They may benefit from learning to interpret physical responses with curiosity rather than fear or shame.

This work is not about teaching a technique alone – it is about restoring trust in the body, one interaction at a time.

OXYTOCIN VS STRESS: THE PRACTICAL GOAL

At the heart of trauma-informed lactation support is a simple neurobiological truth: when oxytocin rises, stress falls.[66]

Oxytocin supports milk ejection, bonding, and emotional regulation. Cortisol, by contrast, inhibits milk flow and heightens anxiety. Many trauma survivors live with chronically elevated stress hormones due to long-standing nervous system activation. This imbalance can interfere with both lactation physiology and emotional availability.

By intentionally supporting oxytocin release, we support not only milk production but also emotional safety and regulation.

In practice, this means:

- Creating moments of emotional safety
- Building predictability into care
- Offering touch only with explicit consent
- Making the feeding environment quiet, private, and supportive
- Reflecting the mother's strengths and intentions
- Celebrating small wins - *"You and your baby are finding your rhythm, even when it feels messy."*

Even when breastfeeding is imperfect, mixed, or short-lived, these oxytocin-rich moments matter. They are not only physiological - they are reparative.

ENSURING SAFETY: THE CLINICAL FOUNDATION

Safety is a prerequisite for oxytocin release, emotional regulation, and learning.[66] For many trauma survivors, bodily autonomy has been historically compromised. Re-establishing agency is therefore not a courtesy — it is therapeutic.

Remind mothers that they are in charge and in control—this may be a new and empowering concept for many survivors.

- *Empower Choice:* Always ask permission before touching. "Would you be comfortable if I touch your breast?" can be a powerful way to return agency.

- *Create Safe Environments:* Consider who is in the room and encourage mothers to ask others to leave if needed. Some may only feel safe breastfeeding when alone or with trusted individuals.
- *Hands-off Techniques:* Practice keeping your hands behind your back and talking through latch adjustments. Online consults can sharpen this skill. However, if hands-on help is essential, always ask first, and be explicit with what you would like to do. Rather than saying "Can I help you?", say "Would it be okay if I touch your breast?"
- *Anchoring Presence:* As a mother once said to me, "She didn't need to know my story, her wholesome presence was enough to get me through that birth." Being present and kind can be profoundly grounding.

This is a powerful reflection of trauma informed care and ensuring safety:

"My body carries memory, seemingly at a cellular level. As I lay on my back, waiting for my baby to be born, the past kept coming back through me but with no context. I was not 'flashing back', I was living in multiple planes of time. My view of reality had been broken right open. I was holding against memories that I couldn't touch or control, and my whole body felt stuck trying to push against it. It's like I was trying to hold my past back behind a dam wall. And yet, I had to get this baby out. My midwife didn't even know my past, but she gently pulled me back into the present, back into the here and now. She was my anchor when I felt like a ship bobbing in the ocean. What I loved about her – she didn't need to know, it was simply her wholesome presence that got me through that birth."

Hands-off lactation support, where feasible, reinforces agency and reduces inadvertent re-enactment of powerlessness. When hands-on assistance is clinically necessary, consent should be specific, ongoing, and revocable, rather than implied.[7]

A consistent theme in trauma literature is that relational safety itself can be healing, even in the absence of trauma disclosure.[73] *Parents do not need to* tell their story to benefit from trauma-informed care — they need to feel respected, anchored, and safe in the present moment.

GENTLE SCREENING WITHOUT DISCLOSURE

Many parents will not disclose a trauma history, and many may not consciously link their feeding distress to past experiences. Trauma-informed care therefore does not rely on direct questioning about trauma. Instead, it relies on noticing, inviting, and creating space for parents to describe their experience in their own terms.

Early in the consultation, gentle, open prompts can help identify when feeding is activating the nervous system without requiring personal disclosure:

- *"Sometimes feeding brings up unexpected feelings for parents. Has anything about breastfeeding felt harder than you expected in a way that's difficult to explain?"*
- *"Do you ever notice feeling tense, shut down, or overwhelmed during feeds?"*
- *"Is there anything I can do to make feeding support feel safer or more comfortable for you?"*
- *"Are there parts of feeding that you find yourself dreading?"*

These questions focus on the present experience rather than the past story. They signal to the parent that their emotional and bodily responses are relevant and welcome in the clinical conversation.

HYPERVIGILANCE AND LACTATION

Hypervigilance is a hallmark of trauma, particularly developmental or repeated trauma. It reflects a state of persistent, heightened alertness in which the nervous system remains on guard for threat. While originally protective, hypervigilance can become exhausting and maladaptive in environments that are no longer dangerous.

In the perinatal period, hypervigilance may present as:

- Constant scanning of the baby's cues
- Difficulty relaxing or sleeping
- Physical tension during feeds
- Intrusive thoughts or fears of "getting it wrong"
- Intense control over feeding schedules, routines, or hygiene

For some, vigilance is expressed outwardly through checking, tracking, and seeking reassurance. For others, it is more internal – emotional rigidity, withdrawal, or dissociation. Hypervigilance may interfere with oxytocin release, reduce milk flow, and make feeding feel unsafe or effortful.

Research has demonstrated that women with trauma histories have significantly higher rates of perinatal PTSD symptoms, anxiety, and physiological stress responses, all of which can influence feeding experiences.[61]

When we understand hypervigilance as protective rather than pathological, we can respond with compassion. The goal is not to eliminate vigilance, but to widen the mother's window of tolerance, allowing moments of safety and connection to emerge alongside necessary alertness.

COPING WITH HYPERVIGILANCE: PRACTICAL STRATEGIES

For Mothers/Parents

- Encourage self-awareness without judgment: *"When you're feeding, what do you notice in your body?"*
- Teach grounding techniques such as slow breathing, sensory anchoring, or mindful pauses
- Validate protective behaviours: *"It makes sense that you're watching things so closely – you're doing your best to keep your baby safe."*
- Support body-based healing if desired, including walking, stretching, yoga, or trauma-informed physiotherapy

- Normalise boundaries with baby – it is okay to need space, to feel touched-out, or to pause feeding

For Providers

- Respond gently even without disclosure – compassion does not require a trauma history
- Adjust physical touch: always ask before assisting with latch or positioning, and offer alternatives such as demonstration or verbal guidance
- Simplify and slow down – trauma survivors are easily overwhelmed by excess information
- Model calm regulation through your tone, pace, and presence
- Normalise feeding behaviour and infant variability to reduce self-blame
- Refer when appropriate – trauma healing often requires multidisciplinary support

Many trauma survivors minimise their experiences, saying, "I didn't have it as bad as others." This self-minimisation is itself a trauma response. It does not mean they are coping – it means they do not believe they deserve care.

Remind them that they do. Every time.

CLOSING: GENTLE CARE FOR TENDER PLACES

Trauma-informed lactation support is not about having all the answers. It is about showing up with humility, empathy, and flexibility.

With the right support, feeding can become more than nourishment. It can become a place of restoration – where the body slowly becomes safer, trust is rebuilt, and long-standing cycles of trauma begin to soften.

With the right support, feeding can become more than nourishment. It can become a place of restoration – where the body slowly becomes safer, trust is rebuilt, and long-standing cycles of trauma begin to soften.

While understanding trauma is essential, insight alone is rarely enough. Many parents need practical tools to help them navigate anxiety, distress, avoidance, intrusive thoughts, hypervigilance, and the emotional challenges that can arise during feeding and early parenting. The next chapter explores a range of evidence-informed strategies, including Acceptance and Commitment Therapy (ACT), Cognitive Behavioural Therapy (CBT), and other supportive approaches that can be integrated into breastfeeding care. These tools are not designed to treat trauma itself, but they can help parents build coping skills, increase psychological flexibility, and create space for feeding relationships to feel safer and more manageable.

REFERENCES

7 Callanan F, Bradshaw C, Tuohy T, Noonan M, Murphy S, Grealish A. An integrative review of how midwives are screening and assessing for trauma in women within perinatal services. PLoS One. 2025;20(7):e0327253.

61 Seng JS, Low LK, Sperlich M, Ronis DL, Liberzon I. Prevalence, trauma history, and risk for posttraumatic stress disorder among nulliparous women in maternity care. Obstet Gynecol. 2009;114(4):839–47.

66 Kendall-Tackett K. Psychological Trauma and Breastfeeding: What We Know So Far. Medical Research Archives. 2022;10.

73 Levine PA. In an Unspoken Voice: How the Body Releases Trauma and Restores Goodness. Berkeley: North Atlantic Books; 2010.

75 van der Kolk B. The Body Keeps the Score: Brain, Mind, and Body in the Healing of Trauma. New York: Viking; 2014.

CHAPTER 10:

Integrating Trauma-Informed Care into Practical Breastfeeding Support

"Between stimulus and response there is a space. In that space is our power to choose our response."

~ Viktor Frankl

As breastfeeding medicine providers, we support families navigating not only the physiology of lactation, but also the emotional and neurobiological sequelae of trauma. This chapter translates trauma-informed principles into practical, evidence-based breastfeeding support, offering concrete strategies that can be integrated into everyday clinical care to enhance safety, agency, and connection.

A growing evidence base supports the integration of trauma-informed approaches across perinatal and lactation care. Recent systematic reviews, qualitative studies, and observational research link traumatic birth and birth-related post-traumatic stress symptoms with reduced breastfeeding initiation, shorter duration, lower maternal self-efficacy, and increased feeding-related distress.[7, 22, 66, 68, 73] These findings highlight the need for early, psychologically attuned lactation support rather than reliance on "standard" advice alone.

At a systems level, qualitative and service-level research demonstrates that trauma-informed practice is strengthened by continuity of care, respectful consent processes, and interprofessional collaboration across midwifery, lactation, psychology/psychiatry, and primary care, while gaps persist in routine screening, staff training, and consistent referral pathways.[7, 67, 68] Together, these findings reinforce what many clinicians already recognise: trauma-informed breastfeeding care is not a niche skill, but a core competency for improving both feeding outcomes and maternal wellbeing.

Trauma-informed care does not require specialist psychotherapy skills. It requires attentiveness to power, consent, predictability, and nervous system regulation — principles that are already central to good breastfeeding medicine practice.[66]

IDENTIFYING TRIGGERS IN BREASTFEEDING CARE

Pregnancy, birth, and breastfeeding involve bodily exposure, sensation, and loss of control — all common trauma cues.[68] Triggers are not pathological; they represent learned survival responses shaped by earlier experiences.

Common breastfeeding-related triggers include:

- Unexpected touch or repositioning
- Pelvic or breast pain
- Infant behaviours such as twiddling or vigorous suckling
- Night-time feeds, fatigue, and sensory overload - sometimes darkenss and fatigue can amplify feelings of vulnerability
- The act of latching itself, especially if it involves unexpected or intense sensations
- Language that implies performance, compliance, or failure

Trauma may alter pain perception and sensory processing through dysregulated stress pathways.[67] When breastfeeding pain appears disproportionate, persistent, or treatment-resistant, trauma should be considered as a contributing factor — not as a dismissal of symptoms, but as part of a broader biopsychosocial and transdiagnostic formulation.

Short-term trigger diaries can assist in identifying patterns and guiding adaptive care without requiring trauma disclosure.

MODIFYING TRIGGERS: ADAPTIVE, COMPASSIONATE CARE

Trauma-informed breastfeeding care prioritises function over ideology. What supports regulation and connection for one parent may be intolerable for another.

Our goal is to make breastfeeding as comfortable as possible, while respecting each mother's autonomy and limits. Some strategies may feel counterintuitive, or quite different to any of the advice you would usually give, but they can make a significant difference.

Adjust the Feeding Environment

- If skin-to-skin contact feels overwhelming, add a layer of clothing or use alternate positions that reduce intense physical closeness.

- Change the room, lighting, or seating arrangements — sometimes small environmental shifts can help.

Support Alternative Feeding Plans

If night-time feeds are a trigger, consider:

- Pumping and offering EBM at night
- Having another caregiver attend to the baby (with the mother's consent and comfort)
- Offering supplemental feeds overnight
- Exploring scheduled feeds to give the mother a sense of control

Reduce Negative Sensory Stimuli

- Try a feeding necklace or bracelet to give the baby something else to hold instead of the mother's skin.
- Offer a substitute, like holding the baby's hand, to reduce twiddling or grabbing.
- Consider nipple shields if they help reduce sensation or discomfort on the nipple.
- Explore if pumping feels safer or easier than direct breastfeeding, and if so, counsel extensively to support informed decision-making, as this is certainly not an easy alternative.

The Power of Permission

Perhaps the most important intervention is offering permission to stop or adjust. One mother said it best:

"Wow, thank you. Nobody has ever given me permission to do that before."

Sometimes, the simple act of saying "It's okay to take a break" or "You can stop if it feels too much" can be the most healing support we can offer.

Offering explicit permission to pause, modify, or stop breastfeeding — without withdrawal of care or support — is frequently described by survivors as profoundly reparative.[66]

INCLUDING PARTNERS AND SUPPORT PEOPLE

Partners and support people can play a powerful role in creating safety during feeding, particularly when trauma triggers are present. With the parent's permission, brief education for partners can transform the feeding environment.

Partners can assist by:

- Adjusting lighting, noise, and privacy
- Helping the parent maintain preferred positioning or clothing layers
- Offering grounding cues such as a hand to hold, a drink of water, or quiet reassurance
- Understanding why phrases such as "just push through" or "let's just give the baby bottles" may be invalidating

When partners understand that feeding distress is a nervous system response rather than a lack of effort, they are more able to support regulation rather than inadvertently increasing pressure.

EDUCATING ABOUT WHAT IS NORMAL

Unmet expectations are a major driver of shame and self-blame in breastfeeding parents.[69] Normalising struggle is therefore a clinical intervention.

Supporting mothers through breastfeeding after trauma — or even in the absence of trauma — requires a deep understanding of the emotional and sensory landscape of feeding. Breastfeeding is not just a biological act; it is an experience shaped by personal history, cultural narratives, and societal expectations. By addressing these factors head-on, we can help mothers feel more at ease in their feeding journeys.

Key educational priorities include:

- Variability in infant feeding behaviour
- The normalcy of cluster feeding and unsettled periods
- The bidirectional relationship between stress and milk ejection
- The distinction between feeding success and parental worth

Normalise the Experience

Breastfeeding can be hard. Many mothers, regardless of their trauma history, struggle with latch, milk supply, pain, fatigue, and feelings of overwhelm. It's important to remind mothers that struggling with breastfeeding is not a failure — it is a common experience, and they are not alone. Peer support groups, breastfeeding counsellors, and lactation professionals can offer vital reassurance and practical tips. Normalising these challenges helps mothers feel less isolated and reduces the pressure to "get it perfect."

As one mother said:

> *"I thought breastfeeding would be natural, but it felt so hard and lonely at times. Knowing that others found it hard too made me feel less like I was doing it wrong."*

Biologic Reframing of the Breast

For some trauma survivors, particularly those with histories of sexual abuse, reframing the breast as an organ of nourishment rather than sexuality can reduce distress and cognitive dissonance.[76] This reframing should always be optional, contextual, and patient-led — but when it resonates, it may restore bodily coherence.

Sensual sensations during breastfeeding, including pleasure, are a normal consequence of oxytocin release and sensory stimulation and do not imply sexual intent.[77] Normalisation without amplification helps reduce shame while respecting boundaries.

The cultural overlay of breasts as sexual objects can create discomfort, confusion, or even distress. It is important to gently reframe the role of the breasts in the context of nourishment and nurturing. Clinicians can affirm that:

- The primary function of the breast is to feed and nurture
- Any associations with sexuality are culturally constructed, not biologically inherent
- The act of breastfeeding does not define or diminish a mother's sexual identity; it is simply a normal, biologic process

This framing can help shift the internal narrative for mothers who feel discomfort, allowing them to view their bodies with compassion and purpose.

A script example that you could use might sound something like this:

"For some women, changing their relationship with their breasts is helpful. It is hard in our culture to not see breasts as sexual. But for now, perhaps you could experiment with your thoughts, and try seeing your breasts as something different. For this chapter of your life, they are not sexual. They are your baby's feeding place. If it is possible in your relationship, and something that speaks to you, some Mums find it helpful not to include their breasts in sexual relations whilst feeding. By keeping breasts solely for breastfeeding, their role and function, and eventually our relationship with our breasts, can change. It is of course helpful if your partner is onboard and understanding about this, is it something you could discuss together privately?"

This gives the mother permission to take ownership of her body and how it is used during this chapter. She may not have considered this as an option, and it also puts no pressure on her to discuss this in front of you.

GROUNDING, IMAGERY, AND MINDFULNESS

Grounding strategies are first-line tools for managing dissociation and affective flooding in clinical settings.[49] These techniques are brief, practical, and compatible with breastfeeding. These techniques are particularly useful when clients experience flooding, dissociation, or overwhelming emotions. The goal is short-term – to bring the person back to the present moment.

Sensory Grounding Exercise

Help the parent name:
5 things they can see
4 things they can touch
3 things they can hear
2 things they can smell
1 thing they can taste

Script: *"Let's take a moment. Look around the room. Can you tell me five things you see? Now, four things you can touch... Keep going until we reach one thing you can taste. How do you feel now?"*

Guided Imagery

Invite the parent to visualise a safe space. Use metaphors such as a walk into a peaceful forest, or placing difficult memories inside a secure vault. This helps shift attention away from distressing thoughts.

Script: *"Picture a vault—heavy, solid, safe. Imagine placing the memory or feeling that is bothering you into that vault. Close the door. Lock it. Now gently walk away, leaving it behind. You are safe."*

Breathing Techniques

Teach the 5-5-6 method: Inhale for 5 seconds, hold for 5, exhale for 6. Alternatively, box breathing (inhale, hold, exhale, hold—all for 4 counts) works well.

Transitional Objects

These are tangible items that help a person stay anchored during emotional distress. They serve as physical reminders of strength, safety, or supportive messages.

- Examples include a smooth stone from a beach where they felt calm, a bracelet received during a significant moment, a printed affirmation card, a necklace, or a fidget ring.
- Encourage clients to choose something small, comforting, and portable — something that "brings them back."
- Suggestion: "Could you carry a small item that makes you feel safe or reminds you of how far you've come? You might hold it during feeds or when things feel overwhelming."

Pre-recorded Tools

Recommend apps, YouTube videos, or websites offering calming scripts or mindfulness recordings. Repeated listening often increases effectiveness. Consider preparing a list of vetted resources to share.

These strategies are regulation tools, not trauma-processing interventions.

There are further suggestions and resources in the Appendices of this book.

5-4-3-2-1
GROUNDING METHOD

5 — **5 THINGS YOU CAN SEE**
Look around and notice five things you can see.

4 — **4 THINGS YOU CAN FEEL**
Notice four things you can feel (touch, texture, temperature).

3 — **3 THINGS YOU CAN HEAR**
Listen and notice three things you can hear.

2 — **2 THINGS YOU CAN SMELL**
Notice two things you can smell.

1 — **1 THING YOU CAN TASTE**
Notice one thing you can taste.

TAKE A SLOW BREATH.
YOU ARE HERE. YOU ARE SAFE.

RHYTHM AS REGULATION

Rhythm supports autonomic regulation through predictability and repetition.[78] Gentle movement, rocking, tapping, chewing, or humming can assist both parent and infant in down-regulating arousal.

Movement-based and expressive therapies (e.g. yoga, walking, swimming, dance) support somatic integration and may be particularly helpful for trauma-affected parents seeking non-verbal pathways to reconnection.[76]

Body Movement

Movement is inherently regulating. The gentle sway of rocking, the repetitive motion of walking, or the fluid grace of dancing all help discharge stress and release built-up tension. Encouraging mothers to explore rhythmic body movements — whether it's sitting on a fitball and gently bouncing, pacing the room with the baby in a carrier, or swaying side to side while holding their infant — can soothe both mother and baby. Movement also supports lymphatic flow, reduces muscular tension, and releases endorphins — the body's natural mood boosters.

Even small movements can help. For a mother feeling "stuck" in a chair during a feed, suggesting she gently rock her feet on the floor, sway her shoulders, or softly hum a rhythm can restore a sense of agency and ease.

Chewing or Tapping

For some, rhythmic oral or tactile stimulation offers a powerful way to reorient the mind and soothe the body. Chewing gum, sucking on a lozenge, or even rhythmically chewing food can activate the parasympathetic nervous system and signal safety to the brain. Similarly, tapping techniques — like tapping the fingers on the table, drumming on the knees, or using the Emotional Freedom Technique (EFT) to tap acupressure points — can redirect focus from overwhelming sensations and promote a sense of grounding.

These small, subtle strategies are especially helpful during breastfeeding sessions when mothers might feel overwhelmed but need to stay seated or stationary.

Expressive Therapies

Rhythmic expression through dance, sport, and other nonverbal activities offers another avenue for healing. Trauma often disconnects people from their bodies, creating a sense of detachment or even distrust. Engaging in movement-based practices like yoga, martial arts, swimming, or expressive dance helps mothers reconnect with their bodies in a way that feels safe, strong, and free. For some, running or cycling provides a release; for others, it might be as simple as swaying to music in the kitchen.

These forms of nonverbal expression are not just hobbies or pastimes — they are therapeutic tools that can help mothers process complex emotions without needing to find the words. They create opportunities for rhythm, flow, and pleasure — elements that trauma can often strip away.

COGNITIVE BEHAVIOURAL THERAPY (CBT): PRACTICAL INTEGRATION

Cognitive Behavioural Therapy (CBT) is a practical, evidence-based approach for perinatal anxiety and depression, and it can be especially helpful when trauma has left a mother with loud inner criticism, catastrophic predictions, and a sense of failure that intensifies during feeding.[14] The heart of CBT is learning to notice thoughts (and the meanings we attach to sensations), and then gently testing whether those thoughts are accurate, useful, and compassionate. This is especially important for mothers in the perinatal period, when sleep deprivation, hormonal shifts, and social pressures can amplify negative self-talk and fuel anxiety or feelings of inadequacy.

Two trauma-informed principles matter here:

1. we do not argue with a mother's fear
2. we widen her options for responding to it

CBT is not about "positive thinking." It is about accurate thinking under stress.

CBT IN TRAUMA-INFORMED BREASTFEEDING SUPPORT: WHAT IT LOOKS LIKE

1. Catch the thought in real time (micro-CBT)

Many mothers cannot sit down and do worksheets in the early postpartum period. A simple adaptation is to capture thoughts in the phone or on a notepad (notes app or a voice memo). The goal is not to solve it immediately; it's to stop the thought from becoming the atmosphere. This also works as a thought journal which you can discuss together in a future consult to fact-check the accuracy of the thoughts.

Prompt you can offer:

- "If your mind says something sharp during a feed, can you jot a few words down? Just enough to catch it."

Common examples:

- "I'm starving her."
- "She hates breastfeeding."
- "My body is failing."
- "I can't do this."
- "I'm a bad mother."

2. Name the pattern (without pathologising it)

Help her see the mind doing what minds do under threat: predicting danger, scanning for failure, trying to prevent shame.

You might say:

- "Your brain is trying to protect you by preparing for the worst. That's a very understandable response when you have a little human who depends entirely on you."

3. Test the thought with gentle, concrete evidence

Use the baby's data and the mother's lived observations. Keep it small and specific.

Questions:

- "What makes you think that's true?"
- "What would we expect to see if it were true?"
- "What evidence do we have today that points the other way?"

Examples:

- If the thought is "I'm starving her," look at weight gain, output, swallowing, satiety cues, and the overall pattern — not one difficult feed.
- If the thought is "I can't do this," explore what she has already done: "You got through the last 24 hours. What helped, even a little?"

4. Reframe into something truer, kinder, and actionable.

Reframes should feel believable. They should also create a next step.

Examples:

- "I'm starving her" → "I'm anxious because feeding is hard; today the signs suggest she is getting milk."
- "My body is failing" → "My body is under stress; we can support supply and reduce pressure."
- "I'm a bad mother" → "I'm overwhelmed and still showing up."

5. Use a brief 'stop and shift' tool for repetitive self-attack, such as visualisation:

- Picture a bright red stop sign.
- Pair with: "This is a thought, not a fact."
- Then add a grounding action: feel feet on floor, soften shoulders, exhale longer than inhale.

This sequence matters: **interrupt → label → regulate.**

Like muscle memory, the more frequently this intervention is applied, the easier it becomes, and the disruptive or distressing thoughts are able to be halted with increasing ease.

6. Add a body-based CBT tool: Progressive Muscle Relaxation (PMR)

PMR is useful because trauma often lives as muscle tension. A mother can do a 30–60 second PMR during a feed without anyone noticing: unclench jaw, drop shoulders, open hands.

Clinician script:

- *"Let's try one tiny experiment. As your baby latches, can you soften your shoulders by 10% and unclench your jaw? Not perfect — just a little."*

This builds self-efficacy: *"I can influence what happens in my body."*

For a longer version of PMR, please see the information box on the next page.

7. Keep CBT from becoming another perfection project

For trauma-affected mothers, CBT can become "homework that I failed." Keep it light:

- one thought
- one reframe
- one body cue

That is enough.
The goal is not forced positivity, but cognitive flexibility.

PROGRESSIVE MUSCLE RELAXATION (PMR) SCRIPT

1 GROUNDING AND BREATH

- Find a comfortable position (sitting or lying down).
- Close your eyes or soften your gaze.
- Take a slow, deep breath in... and gently release it.
- Repeat this slow, steady breathing, noticing the support of the ground or chair beneath you.

2 PROGRESSIVE MUSCLE RELAXATION

Hands and Arms

- Clench your fists, hold briefly, then release.
- Tighten your forearms and upper arms, hold, then release.

Feet and Legs

- Curl your toes downward, hold, then release.
- Tighten your calves and thighs, hold, then release.

Face and Jaw

- Scrunch your face (wrinkle forehead, close eyes, clench jaw), hold, then release.
- Allow your jaw to soften and your forehead to smooth.

Shoulders and Neck

- Lift your shoulders towards your ears, hold, then release.
- Let your shoulders settle downwards.

Torso and Back

- Tighten your stomach muscles, hold, then release.
- Allow your back to soften against the support beneath you.

3 FULL BODY SCAN

- Take a moment to scan your body from head to toe.
- Notice any areas of lingering tension.
- Invite these areas to soften with each out-breath.
- It is normal for some tension to remain; the practice encourages gentle awareness, not perfection.

4 CLOSING

- Take a few comfortable breaths, noticing how your body feels now.
- Gently wiggle your fingers and toes.
- When ready, open your eyes or lift your gaze.
- Take a moment to acknowledge your body and its efforts today.

TAKE A SLOW BREATH.
YOU ARE HERE. YOU ARE SAFE.

ACCEPTANCE AND COMMITMENT THERAPY (ACT): VALUES-BASED CARE

ACT is often an ideal fit for breastfeeding in the context of trauma because it does not demand that distress disappears before a mother can feed her baby or bond. ACT teaches that difficult thoughts and feelings can be present, and she can still choose actions aligned with her values.[79]

This matters in trauma because the nervous system may react even when the mother logically "knows" she is safe. ACT respects that reality.

ACT IN BREASTFEEDING SUPPORT: THE CORE STEPS

1. Values: return to what matters (the Values Compass)

A rigid goal (exclusive breastfeeding at all costs) can become a trauma amplifier. Values give a wider, kinder target.

Questions:

- "What kind of mother do you want to be in feeding moments?"
- "When you look back on this season, what do you hope your baby felt?"

Common values: nurturing, steadiness, protection, tenderness, presence, flexibility, dignity.

Values-based reframe:

- "The goal isn't a perfect feed. The goal is a feeding relationship that aligns with care and safety."

2. Replace 'but' with 'and'

This simple shift stops the mind from forcing a single story.

Examples:

- "I want to breastfeed and it brings up a lot."
- "I love my baby and I feel touched-out."
- "This is meaningful and it is hard."

This is emotionally regulating in itself.

3. Cognitive defusion: unhook from the thought

ACT doesn't wrestle the thought; it changes the relationship to it.

Scripts:

- "I'm noticing I'm having the thought that I'm failing."
- "Thank you mind — there's that scary story again."

Imagery options (choose what suits the mother):

- leaves on a stream – the intrusive thoughts can be visualised as leaves that keep on floating past without getting stuck and staying.
- clouds passing - we are the sky and the thoughts are clouds passing through.
- thoughts on a sushi train: "I don't have to pick that one up."

4. Make room for sensation (without flooding)

With trauma, "be present in your body" can be too much. The dose matters. Aim for partial presence.

A graded approach:

- choose one safe anchor (feet on floor, hand on chest, baby's warmth on the forearm)
- stay with it for two breaths
- return to the moment

You can say:

- *"We're not forcing full presence. We're practising tiny, safe contact with the present."*

5. Committed action: one small step that matches values

When the mother is activated, the action should be small enough to be doable.

Examples:

- value: tenderness → “One slow breath before latching.”
- value: dignity → “Asking staff to explain before touching.”
- value: safety → “Choosing a position that feels less exposed.”
- value: presence → “One moment of eye contact mid-feed.”

6. Self-compassion as a clinical intervention

Trauma often installs an internal voice that is harsh and absolute. ACT invites a different stance.

Prompts:

- “If your best friend said this to you, what would you tell her?”
- “Can we try speaking to yourself the way you’d speak to your baby?”

Simple phrases (short, repeatable, believable):

- “This is hard.”
- “I’m allowed to take it one step at a time.”
- “I can be gentle with myself and still be a good mother.”

7. Practical clinician language (ACT-aligned)

By gently guiding mothers through these practices, we help them cultivate a more spacious, accepting relationship with their inner world. Even if breastfeeding remains difficult, they can still experience moments of connection, agency, and love.

Script Example:

"It makes a lot of sense that breastfeeding might bring up some of those painful feelings or memories — especially if your body has been through trauma. You’re not broken, and you’re not alone in this. What you’re feeling is a response to something really hard that your body and mind remember.

Rather than trying to get rid of these thoughts or feelings, let's gently learn to make space for them — without letting them run the show. So when that wave of anxiety or shame shows up during a feed, you might pause, take a slow breath, and notice what's happening: 'I'm feeling tense in my chest,' or 'That memory is here again.' Instead of fighting it, we say, 'There you are,' and bring the focus back to what matters—maybe looking at your baby's face, or reminding yourself why you want to breastfeed, even though it's hard.

We're not trying to make the feelings disappear—we're helping you stay anchored in what's important, even with those feelings present. And we do it step by step, moment by moment. That's the heart of ACT: making room for what's hard, and still choosing what matters to you."

SETTING BOUNDARIES WITH TODDLERS

Breastfeeding a toddler can be a beautiful, rewarding experience — but it can also bring new challenges, especially when mothers feel touched out, overwhelmed, or unsure how to navigate their child's growing independence. For some, it may feel like they *should* be endlessly available — leading to guilt when they feel the need for space.

Helping mothers understand that it is okay to set limits — and that doing so is an act of love, not rejection—can be transformative. Boundaries can honour both the mother's needs and the toddler's emotional development, creating a more sustainable, respectful breastfeeding relationship.

EMPOWER LIMITS

Many mothers don't realise they can set boundaries in breastfeeding. It can feel as if they must continue to feed on demand, no matter how they feel — especially if they've absorbed messages like "Breastfeeding is all or nothing."

Empower mothers to know that it's okay to say no sometimes. It's okay to limit the number, length, or location of feeds. It's okay to decide that *"I don't want to breastfeed right now"* is a valid and loving response.

You might say:
"It's perfectly normal to feel touched out, tired, or in need of space. Breastfeeding is a relationship, and you're allowed to shape it in a way that feels sustainable for you."

This perspective can be a revelation for many mothers — offering permission to care for themselves *and* their child.

PLAYFUL STRATEGIES FOR BOUNDARIES WITH TODDLERS

For toddlers, play is a powerful tool. Using playful strategies can make the process of setting boundaries feel lighter and more positive — for both mother and child.

Some ideas include:

- Countdowns: *"Let's count to 10 while you have a quick milkie, and then we'll be all done!"*
- Rocket Launches: *"Okay, ready to blast off? 10... (cont) 3... 2... 1... Blast Off!"* As the child becomes familiar with this, you can speed up how fast you count down.
- Songs: Singing a simple song can mark the end of a feed and create a predictable rhythm *(e.g., "This is the end of milk time, now it's time to play!")*
- Special Times: Some mothers introduce the idea of *"milk is for bedtime and nap time"*, using clear routines to structure feeds.

These playful strategies help toddlers feel safe and supported, even when limits are introduced. They also help mothers step into their authority with confidence — knowing that boundaries are not about taking love away, but about creating a balanced, sustainable breastfeeding relationship.

DISSOCIATION: RECOGNITION AND RESPECT

Dissociation is a protective response, not a failure.[61] In breastfeeding, it may enable continuation when full presence feels unsafe. Dissociation is a common coping mechanism among trauma survivors — an automatic, protective response to overwhelming internal or external stimuli. The feelings that come up might include feelings of vulnerability, fear, shame, or inadequacy. For many mothers, dissociation may be the only way they can tolerate certain aspects of pregnancy, birth, or breastfeeding. Understanding and working with — not against — this response is an essential part of trauma-informed care.

Recognise It

Many survivors dissociate during breastfeeding as a way to cope with triggers such as physical touch, exposure, or the intense intimacy of feeding. They may describe feeling detached from their body, emotionally numb, mentally checked-out, or as though they are watching themselves from the outside.

Normalise and Validate

Reassure mothers that dissociation is not a failure — it's a learned survival strategy that helped them get through something painful. Naming it can help reduce shame. You might say:

"*It makes sense that your mind developed ways to protect you. Let's look at how those tools are showing up now.*"

Dissociation vs. Dis-identification

In trauma-informed care, it's important to offer alternatives that help a parent stay present without being overwhelmed. One such approach is dis-identification. Unlike dissociation, which disconnects a person from their experience, dis-identification encourages them to observe their thoughts and feelings without becoming fused with them. It's a gentle separation between *who I am and what I am experiencing right now.* This is another aspect of Acceptance and Commitment Therapy (ACT).

For example, rather than automatically believing the painful thought, "I am a bad mother," a mother might learn to say to herself:

"*I'm noticing that I'm having the thought that I'm a bad mother.*"

This shift creates space. It reminds the parent that thoughts are events in the mind, not absolute truths. Dis-identification invites a stance of curiosity and compassion, rather than judgment or avoidance. It allows the parent to stay emotionally connected to their baby while not becoming consumed by their inner distress.

This strategy can be particularly helpful during breastfeeding, where quiet moments may leave space for intrusive thoughts to arise. Instead of trying to push the thoughts away (which can paradoxically make them stronger) or dissociating (which numbs the entire experience), dis-identification invites the mother to gently notice the thought, label it, and return her focus to the present — the feel of her baby's body against hers, the rhythm of the suckling, the sound of quiet breaths.

Functional Use vs. Growth-Oriented Support

- If dissociation allows the mother to feed her baby and meet her goals, it may be appropriate to simply acknowledge and support it.
- If the mother expresses a desire to enjoy breastfeeding more, feel more present, or feel less disconnected, then offer gentle tools to support that transition.

Supportive Strategies

- Encourage mothers to notice when and how dissociation occurs. Keeping a log of what was happening before, during, and after the dissociative episode can build insight.
- ACT and grounding techniques can help bring the mother back into the present moment. Encourage sensory grounding, breathing techniques, or transitional objects during feeds.
- For some mothers, distraction (e.g., reading, listening to a podcast, scrolling on their phone) during feeds can be a safer bridge than full presence. This can be an adaptive strategy rather than a failure to bond.

Clinician Framing

You might say:

"*Dissociation has helped you survive something incredibly difficult. You don't have to give up that tool right away. But if you want to feel more connected or present, we can explore other ways to support you. There's no right or wrong way — only what feels safe and helpful for you right now.*"

Be Gentle with Transitions

Moving from dissociation to embodied feeding can be overwhelming. Encourage small steps, such as bringing awareness to one part of the body or engaging just one sense (e.g., feeling baby's feet or hearing their suckling). These are moments of presence, even if fleeting.

Permission to Tolerate Rather Than Enjoy

Some mothers may never come to love breastfeeding — and that's okay. Survival, safety, and tolerating the experience might be the most realistic and compassionate goals.

Healing Is Nonlinear

Fluctuating between dissociation and presence is common. Validate this rather than pushing for a linear trajectory.

Coping mechanisms are survival tools. They may not always be ideal outside trauma, but they deserve respect. The goal is not to erase these responses, but to expand the client's repertoire of options. With time and trust, you can help clients move from mere survival to potential healing.

Through compassion, education, and flexibility, you can walk alongside mothers navigating trauma in their breastfeeding journeys. Sometimes healing doesn't look like perfect attachment or joyful feeds — it looks like surviving, finding small joys, and feeling safe again.

"GOOD ENOUGH" PARENTING

The concept of "good enough" parenting, first articulated by Winnicott, offers a vital counterweight to trauma-driven perfectionism.[80] Secure attachment does not require flawless care, but responsiveness over time. Attuned repair over time, and not perfection, is what builds security in attachment.

In the world of breastfeeding support, we often hear messages about the "best start" and "optimal feeding", and while these ideals can inspire, they can also create an impossible standard, especially for mothers navigating trauma, exhaustion, or mental health challenges.

That's why it's vital to introduce the concept of "good enough" parenting. At its heart, "good enough" parenting acknowledges that perfection is not only impossible, but unnecessary. The power of this idea lies in giving mothers permission to be human — to show up as they are, even when they feel overwhelmed or imperfect.

The concept of “good enough” parenting, first articulated by Winnicott, offers a vital counterweight to trauma-driven perfectionism.[80] Secure attachment does not require flawless care, but responsiveness over time. Attuned repair over time, and not perfection, is what builds security in attachment.

In the world of breastfeeding support, we often hear messages about the “best start” and “optimal feeding”, and while these ideals can inspire, they can also create an impossible standard, especially for mothers navigating trauma, exhaustion, or mental health challenges.

That’s why it’s vital to introduce the concept of “good enough” parenting. At its heart, “good enough” parenting acknowledges that perfection is not only impossible, but unnecessary. The power of this idea lies in giving mothers permission to be human — to show up as they are, even when they feel overwhelmed or imperfect.

For many mothers, this shift can be transformative. It invites them to move away from unrealistic ideals and instead focus on sustainability, presence, and self-compassion.

Realistic Expectations

No breastfeeding journey is flawless. There will be feeds where the baby is fussy, the latch is painful, or emotions run high. By helping mothers develop realistic expectations, we can relieve the pressure of perfectionism.

You might say:

"Not every feed has to be perfect. It’s okay to have moments where things feel messy or hard — what matters is the big picture, not the individual feed."

Encourage mothers to see each feeding session as just one part of the broader tapestry of healing — a journey made up of good days, hard days, and everything in between.

Celebrating Small Victories

In the pursuit of "good enough," it's essential to acknowledge and celebrate small wins. These moments might seem insignificant to others, but for a mother navigating trauma or distress, they can be huge milestones:

- A feed where she felt more present, even for a few minutes.
- A moment where she paused to take a breath before latching.
- A decision to stop and prioritise rest when she needed it.

You might say:

"*That time you took a breath and noticed your baby's eyes during a feed — that was a win.*"

These moments deserve recognition because they build a sense of competence and hope — key ingredients for long-term resilience.

Self-Compassion

Perhaps the most critical skill in "good enough" parenting is learning to treat oneself with kindness. Many mothers hold themselves to harsh standards, comparing themselves to idealised versions of what a "good mother" should be.

Encourage mothers to forgive themselves for moments of struggle—to recognise that frustration, exhaustion, and even ambivalence are part of the human experience.

You might ask:

"*What would you say to a friend who felt like they weren't doing enough?*"

Help mothers see that progress matters more than perfection. Every time they choose to pause, breathe, or show up as best they can, they are building a stronger, more compassionate relationship with themselves and their baby.

"Good enough" parenting does not mean settling for less or giving up on goals. It means recognising that healing is not linear, and that a sustainable, nurturing relationship with a baby is built on flexibility, presence, and forgiveness.

As clinicians, we can remind mothers that their baby doesn't need a perfect parent — they need a parent who is present, responsive, and human. When we help mothers embrace the messy, beautiful reality of "good enough," we create space for growth, healing, and love to flourish.

WHEN ADDITIONAL MENTAL HEALTH SUPPORT IS INDICATED

Trauma-informed breastfeeding care supports regulation and agency, but it is not a substitute for trauma therapy. At times, additional mental health support is necessary.

Consider referral when there is:

- Persistent panic, flashbacks, or intrusive memories during feeds
- An inability to remain present even briefly despite grounding strategies
- Feeding decisions driven primarily by fear, shame, or avoidance
- Severe self-blame, hopelessness, or emotional numbing
- A parent expressing that feeding feels re-traumatising
- Any risk of harm to self or children

Trauma-informed care in these situations can make psychological therapy more accessible by first restoring a sense of safety and control in the feeding relationship.

CLOSING REFLECTIONS

Trauma-informed breastfeeding support is not about perfect technique or ideal outcomes. It is about safety, dignity, and relational repair. Sometimes healing looks like joy. Sometimes it looks like tolerance. Both are valid.

Our role is not to eliminate distress, but to walk alongside parents as they rebuild trust — in their bodies, their babies, and themselves.

ACT-Based Strategies for Supporting Breastfeeding Parents

ACT TOOL	PURPOSE	EXAMPLE
Values Compass	Clarify what matters most as a parent and use these values to guide decisions.	*"What kind of parent do you want to be?"*
Reframing Goals	Shift from rigid feeding goals to values-based intentions.	*"Let's focus on how feeding feels, not just what it looks like."*
Committed Action	Identify small, values-aligned steps that can be taken today.	*"If presence is important to you, could you pause for a breath before a feed?"*
Normalising Conflict	Acknowledge that competing values and emotions can coexist.	*"I want to breastfeed, and I'm finding it hard."*
Cognitive Defusion	Create distance from difficult thoughts rather than arguing with them.	*"There's that thought again."*
Replace 'But' with 'And'	Encourage acceptance of multiple truths at once.	*"I want to breastfeed, and I'm struggling."*
Self-Compassion	Reduce self-criticism and foster kindness towards oneself.	*"What would you say to a friend in this situation?"*
Dis-Identification	Help parents recognise they are not their thoughts.	*"I'm noticing the thought that I'm a bad mother."*
Visualisation	Use imagery to observe thoughts without becoming entangled in them.	*"Imagine the thought floating past on a stream."*
Grounding in the Present	Redirect attention to the current moment and what matters now.	*"Take a slow breath and notice your baby's face."*
Permission to Coexist	Allow difficult emotions while continuing to act according to values.	*"The pain is here, and I can still choose to nurture my baby."*

Adapted from Acceptance and Commitment Therapy (ACT) principles applied to breastfeeding support.

REFERENCES

7 Callanan F, Bradshaw C, Tuohy T, Noonan M, Murphy S, Grealish A. An integrative review of how midwives are screening and assessing for trauma in women within perinatal services. PLoS One. 2025;20(7):e0327253.

22 Cavallé-Abasolo E, Dikmen-Yildiz P, Gómez-Gómez I, Barros-Martins L, Motrico E. Impact of Traumatic Childbirth and Birth-Related Posttraumatic Stress Disorder on Breastfeeding Outcomes: A Systematic Review of Longitudinal and Cohort Studies. Birth. 2025;52(4):553–71.

49 Dekel S, Stuebe C, Dishy G. Childbirth Induced Posttraumatic Stress Syndrome: A Systematic Review of Prevalence and Risk Factors. Front Psychol. 2017;8:560.

61 Seng JS, Low LK, Sperlich M, Ronis DL, Liberzon I. Prevalence, trauma history, and risk for posttraumatic stress disorder among nulliparous women in maternity care. Obstet Gynecol. 2009;114(4):839–47.

66 Kendall-Tackett K. Psychological Trauma and Breastfeeding: What We Know So Far. Medical Research Archives. 2022;10.

67 Moog NK, Buss C, Entringer S, Shahbaba B, Gillen DL, Hobel CJ, et al. Maternal Exposure to Childhood Trauma Is Associated During Pregnancy With Placental-Fetal Stress Physiology. Biol Psychiatry. 2016;79(10):831–9.

68 Beck CT, Watson S. Subsequent childbirth after a previous traumatic birth. Nurs Res. 2010;59(4):241–9.

69 COPE. Mental health care in the perinatal period: Australian clinical practice guideline. Melbourne: Centre of Perinatal Excellence (COPE); 2023.

73 Levine PA. In an Unspoken Voice: How the Body Releases Trauma and Restores Goodness. Berkeley: North Atlantic Books; 2010

76 van der Kolk BA. Clinical implications of neuroscience research in PTSD. Ann N Y Acad Sci. 2006;1071:277–93.

77 Whitley J, Wouk K, Bauer AE, Grewen K, Gottfredson NC, Meltzer-Brody S, et al. Oxytocin during breastfeeding and maternal mood symptoms. Psychoneuroendocrinology. 2020;113:104581.

78 Porges S. The Polyvagal Theory. New York: Norton.

79 Harris R. ACT Made Simple. 2nd ed. Oakland, CA: New Harbinger Publications; 2025.

80 Winnicott DW. Transitional objects and transitional phenomena; a study of the first not-me possession. Int J Psychoanal. 1953;34(2):89–97.

CHAPTER 11:

Holding the Whole Story – A Structured Approach to Trauma-Informed Infant Feeding Care

"The most important thing in communication is hearing what isn't said."

~ Peter Drucker

Supporting infant feeding in the context of trauma is not a linear or protocol-driven task. It requires clinicians to tolerate complexity, hold apparent contradictions, and remain present with vulnerability — often without immediate resolution. Trauma-informed lactation care asks us to attend not only to feeding mechanics, but to meaning, safety, and the relational context in which feeding occurs.[72]

This chapter outlines a structured, integrative framework for trauma-informed infant feeding care. It brings together recognition, inquiry, relational safety, practical intervention, referral pathways, and clinician sustainability — allowing care to be both consistent and deeply individualised.

A STEP-BY-STEP FRAMEWORK FOR TRAUMA-INFORMED INFANT FEEDING SUPPORT

1. Recognition

Trauma-informed care begins with the assumption — supported by population data — that many parents will carry trauma histories, whether disclosed or not.[3] Recognition does not require identification of specific events. It requires an attuned clinical stance.

Key elements include:

- Sensitive intake processes that avoid pathologising language
- Warm curiosity rather than interrogation
- An awareness that feeding distress may be the expression of earlier adversity, not a failure of motivation or skill

Recognition shifts the clinical stance from *"Why isn't this working?"* to *"What might be making this hard right now?"*

2. Inquiry

Inquiry invites narrative without demanding disclosure. Open-ended, neutral questions allow parents to shape the depth and direction of the conversation.[81]

Examples include:

- "How did the birth feel for you?"
- "What has feeding been like so far?"
- "Are there moments that feel particularly difficult or overwhelming?"

When trauma screening tools or validated questionnaires are used, they should be:

- Contextualised
- Optional
- Followed up with care and containment

Screening without capacity for response risks increasing shame rather than safety.[69]

3. Validation

Validation is a core therapeutic intervention. It reduces shame, supports emotional regulation, and strengthens the therapeutic alliance.[72]

Effective validation:

- Names the emotional experience
- Links current distress to understandable responses
- Avoids minimisation or premature reassurance

Statements such as *"It makes sense that this feels hard"* or *"You have been through a lot; your reactions are understandable"* help parents feel seen without being defined by trauma.

4. Safety and Empowerment

Safety — physical, emotional, and relational — is foundational for both trauma recovery and lactation physiology.[66] Empowerment restores agency where it has previously been compromised.

Clinically, this involves:

- Explicit consent before touch
- Choice around positioning, pacing, and feeding methods
- Respect for refusal, hesitation, or ambivalence
- Reinforcement of autonomy, including the option not to breastfeed

Empowerment-oriented language (for example, *"You are in control of this experience"*) supports oxytocin release, reduces stress responses, and strengthens parental self-efficacy.[77]

5. Intervention and Referral

Trauma-informed intervention prioritises regulation before resolution. Appropriate strategies may include:

- Grounding techniques during feeds
- ACT-informed language to reduce cognitive fusion
- Sensory modifications to the feeding environment
- Flexible feeding plans aligned with parental values

Referral to trauma-informed mental health professionals is indicated when:

- Distress is persistent or escalating
- Dissociation or panic interferes with daily functioning
- Feeding becomes a primary site of re-traumatisation

Warm, relational handover — rather than abrupt referral — preserves trust and continuity of care.[61]

THE TRAUMA-INFORMED FLOW OF A BREASTFEEDING CONSULTATION

Trauma-informed care is not only what we say, but how we structure the consultation. A predictable, respectful flow reduces threat and increases a parent's sense of control.

A helpful sequence is:

1 **ESTABLISH SAFETY AND CONSENT**
- Before any physical contact

2 **OBSERVE BEFORE INTERVENING**
- Pause, watch, understand

3 **ASK BEFORE SUGGESTING**
- Invite collaboration, not correction

4 **NORMALISE BEFORE EDUCATING**
- Reduce shame, create openness

5 **OFFER OPTIONS BEFORE CREATING A PLAN**
- Support autonomy and choice

6 **END BY REINFORCING THE PARENT'S AGENCY AND STRENGTHS**
- Reflect back what is working

This sequence slows the clinician down in a way that is regulating for the parent. It shifts the consultation from expert-led to collaborative, without sacrificing clinical effectiveness.

CREATING A COLLABORATIVE, MULTIDISCIPLINARY SUPPORT SYSTEM

Trauma-informed infant feeding care does not exist in isolation. Outcomes are optimised when clinicians work within collaborative, non-hierarchical systems.

Key components include:

Lactation and Mental Health Collaboration

- Shared language, mutual respect, and aligned goals reduce fragmentation of care.[66]

Peer Support Networks

- Connection with others who share lived experience reduces isolation and normalises struggle.[82]

Ongoing Professional Development

- Training in trauma-informed practice, somatic awareness, attachment theory, and cultural humility strengthens clinical confidence and reduces inadvertent harm.[72]

PREVENTING VICARIOUS TRAUMA: CARING FOR THE CLINICIAN

Trauma-informed work is meaningful — and cumulative. Without adequate support, clinicians are at risk of burnout, compassion fatigue, and vicarious trauma.[83] Vicarious trauma represents a shift in worldview that occurs when professionals repeatedly engage empathetically with trauma survivors, fundamentally altering beliefs about safety and justice in the world. This differs from compassion fatigue, which is a reduced capacity for empathy as a self-protective mechanism following single or cumulative trauma exposure.[84]

Protective strategies include:

- Regular supervision and reflective practice
- Attention to bodily regulation and rest
- Clear professional boundaries and referral pathways
- Recognition that presence does not require perfection

Clinician wellbeing is not ancillary to trauma-informed care — it is integral to it.

CLOSING REFLECTIONS: HOLDING THE WHOLE STORY

Trauma-informed infant feeding care may involve skilled clinical intervention, or it may involve quiet witnessing. Often, it is simply making space for a parent to say, *"This is hard."*

Our role is not to fix, persuade, or override.
It is to accompany — with steadiness, humility, and compassion.

To hold the whole story.

And to remind every mother, quietly and consistently:
She is not alone.

REFERENCES

3 Felitti VJ, Anda RF, Nordenberg D, Williamson DF, Spitz AM, Edwards V, et al. Relationship of childhood abuse and household dysfunction to many of the leading causes of death in adults. The Adverse Childhood Experiences (ACE) Study. Am J Prev Med. 1998;14(4):245–58.

61 Seng JS, Low LK, Sperlich M, Ronis DL, Liberzon I. Prevalence, trauma history, and risk for posttraumatic stress disorder among nulliparous women in maternity care. Obstet Gynecol. 2009;114(4):839–47.

66 Kendall-Tackett K. Psychological Trauma and Breastfeeding: What We Know So Far. Medical Research Archives. 2022;10.

69 COPE. Mental health care in the perinatal period: Australian clinical practice guideline. Melbourne: Centre of Perinatal Excellence (COPE); 2023.
7

72 SAMHSA. SAMHSA's Concept of Trauma and Guidance for a Trauma-Informed Approach. Rockville, MD; 2014. Report No.: (SMA) 14-4884.

77 Whitley J, Wouk K, Bauer AE, Grewen K, Gottfredson NC, Meltzer-Brody S, et al. Oxytocin during breastfeeding and maternal mood symptoms. Psychoneuroendocrinology. 2020;113:104581.

81 Beck CT. Birth trauma: in the eye of the beholder. Nurs Res. 2004;53(1):28–35.

82 Dennis CL. Peer support within a health care context: a concept analysis. Int J Nurs Stud. 2003;40(3):321–32.

83 Ravi A, Gorelick J, Pal H. Identifying and Addressing Vicarious Trauma. Am Fam Physician. 2021;103(9):570–2.

84 Forkey H, Szilagyi M, Kelly ET, Duffee J, THE COUNCIL ON FOSTER CARE A, KINSHIP CARE COCP, COUNCIL ON CHILD ABUSE, et al. Trauma-Informed Care. Pediatrics. 2021;148(2).

84 Forkey H, Szilagyi M, Kelly ET, Duffee J, THE COUNCIL ON FOSTER CARE A, KINSHIP CARE COCP, COUNCIL ON CHILD ABUSE, et al. Trauma-Informed Care. Pediatrics. 2021;148(2).

CHAPTER 12:

Caring, Not Curing – Closing Reflections on Trauma-Informed Breastfeeding Support

"To truly listen is to risk being changed by what we hear."

~ Mark Nepo

As this resource draws to a close, we return to the central premise of trauma-informed breastfeeding care: humility, partnership, and compassion. Our role is not to fix, correct, or resolve a person's past. It is to walk alongside — with skill, curiosity, and respect — in a profoundly vulnerable season of life.

Trauma-informed care does not ask clinicians to become therapists. It asks us to practise medicine, lactation care, and support in ways that prioritise safety, dignity, and agency. When this is done well, care itself can be therapeutic — even in the absence of formal psychotherapy.

This chapter distils key principles into practical reminders for everyday clinical practice — for the families we serve, and for ourselves.

CORE CLINICAL REMINDERS

Individualise Every Plan

There is no universal breastfeeding pathway. Trauma-informed care requires that feeding plans are co-created, revisited, and adapted over time. What is supportive in one season may feel overwhelming in another. Flexibility is not a compromise of care — it is a hallmark of it.[72]

Let Her Be Your Guide

The clinician's role is not to direct, but to support. Ask what breastfeeding means to her, what she hopes for, and what feels possible right now. Honour her stated goals, even when they differ from professional ideals or population-level recommendations.

Meet Her Where She Is

Trust develops slowly for many trauma-affected mothers. Go at her pace. Adjust your language, your presence, and your expectations with care.

Trauma-informed practice is relational — it unfolds over time, not through urgency or pressure.[81]

Remember That "Good Enough" Is Enough

Success is not defined by exclusivity, duration, or technical perfection. Reflective capacity, emotional safety, and secure attachment can develop within a wide range of feeding experiences. A feeding journey does not need to be flawless to be meaningful.[80]

Breastfeeding Can Be Healing — But It Is Not Mandatory

When breastfeeding aligns with a mother's values and feels emotionally tolerable, it may support mental health, bodily trust, and relational repair.[8]

When it does not, stepping away may be protective rather than harmful. Both pathways deserve respect.

IF YOU ARE UNSURE, CONSIDER TRAUMA

Some mothers present with feeding difficulties that feel disproportionate, confusing, or resistant to standard intervention. Others present with known trauma histories that are reactivated by the stress, intimacy, and exposure inherent in infant feeding.

Mental health and breastfeeding are deeply interconnected. When one is under strain, the other often follows. Trauma history does not predict breastfeeding failure — but awareness of trauma allows clinicians to contextualise distress with empathy rather than judgement.[50]

When something feels missing, unexplained, or out of proportion — pause.
Consider trauma.
Then listen.

WHEN YOU ARE THE ONE CARRYING THE WEIGHT

Trauma-informed work is meaningful, relational, and often deeply moving. It can also be heavy. Vicarious trauma and emotional fatigue are real, and they do not reflect personal weakness or professional inadequacy.[83]

Prioritise your own wellbeing

What arises in you during this work matters. Reflection, supervision, and peer support are essential for sustainability. Clinician wellbeing is not optional — it directly shapes the quality of care we provide.

Burnout Is Not a Badge of Honour

You do not need to do everything yourself. Refer when needed. Share care. Rest without apology. Trauma-informed care is best delivered within networks, not in isolation.

Find and Nurture Your Circle

Cultivate a group of trusted colleagues — lactation professionals, mental health clinicians, GPs, midwives — with whom you can collaborate, refer, and debrief.

Supervision Is an Act of Self-Respect

Clinical supervision supports growth, perspective, and emotional containment. It helps preserve not only competence, but compassion.

CLOSING REFLECTIONS

Some mothers want to breastfeed — and with the right support, they can. Find those mothers and offer them everything you can.

Others may choose not to — and that choice, too, deserves care, respect, and affirmation.

There is nothing to rescue.
Nothing to cure.
We don't need to "fix" what somebody has been carrying for a long time.

Our work is to accompany — with steadiness, knowledge, and humility.
To listen.
To reflect back a mother's strength when she forgets it exists.

When bodies are supported to do what they can, and minds are held with care, healing often follows — quietly, imperfectly, and on its own terms.

You are here to care, not cure.
And that is enough.

REFERENCES

8 Kendall-Tackett K, Cong Z, Hale TW. Depression, sleep quality, and maternal well-being in postpartum women with a history of sexual assault: a comparison of breastfeeding, mixed-feeding, and formula-feeding mothers. Breastfeed Med. 2013;8(1):16–22.

50 Wosu AC, Gelaye B, Williams MA. History of childhood sexual abuse and risk of prenatal and postpartum depression or depressive symptoms: an epidemiologic review. Arch Womens Ment Health. 2015;18(5):659–71.

72 SAMHSA. SAMHSA's Concept of Trauma and Guidance for a Trauma-Informed Approach. Rockville, MD; 2014. Report No.: (SMA) 14-4884.

80 Winnicott DW. Transitional objects and transitional phenomena; a study of the first not-me possession. Int J Psychoanal. 1953;34(2):89–97.

81 Beck CT. Birth trauma: in the eye of the beholder. Nurs Res. 2004;53(1):28–35.

83 Ravi A, Gorelick J, Pal H. Identifying and Addressing Vicarious Trauma. Am Fam Physician. 2021;103(9):570–2.

85 Rogers CR. The necessary and sufficient conditions of therapeutic personality change. 1957. J Consult Clin Psychol. 1992;60(6):827–32.

APPENDICES AND FURTHER RESOURCES

APPENDIX A: KNOLEDGE CHECK AND DETAILED ANSWERS

1. *DSM-5 Criteria for PTSD*

Question:
Which of the following is a required criterion for the diagnosis of Posttraumatic Stress Disorder (PTSD) according to DSM-5?

Options:
A. Avoidance of distressing memories, thoughts, or feelings
B. Hypervigilance and exaggerated startle response
C. Exposure to actual or threatened death, serious injury, or sexual violence
D. Persistent negative beliefs or expectations about oneself or the world

Correct Answer: C

Rationale:
According to DSM-5, exposure to actual or threatened death, serious injury, or sexual violence is a necessary criterion for the diagnosis of PTSD. Options A and B represent symptoms within specific symptom clusters, while Option D is part of the "negative alterations in cognitions and mood" cluster.

2. *Outcomes Associated with Adverse Childhood Experiences (ACEs)*

Question:
In the context of Adverse Childhood Experiences (ACEs), what is a common outcome associated with individuals who have experienced multiple ACEs?

Options:

A. Enhanced resilience and stress management skills
B. Lower risk of mental health disorders
C. Increased susceptibility to chronic health conditions
D. Improved academic performance

Correct Answer: C

Rationale:
Research consistently demonstrates that individuals with multiple ACEs have increased risk of chronic physical and mental health conditions in adulthood, including cardiovascular disease, autoimmune illness, depression, and anxiety.

3. *Risk Factors for Birth Trauma*

Question:
Which of the following factors is often associated with an increased risk of birth trauma?

Options:

A. High levels of social support during pregnancy
B. Detailed birth planning with flexible expectations
C. Smooth and uncomplicated labour
D. Lack of control or feelings of powerlessness during childbirth

Correct Answer: D

Rationale:
Perceived loss of control, lack of consent, and feelings of powerlessness are strongly associated with birth trauma, regardless of clinical outcomes.

4. *Triggers for PTSD Related to Breastfeeding*

Question:
For individuals with PTSD related to breastfeeding, which of the following could act as a potential trigger?

Options:
A. A supportive and understanding breastfeeding environment
B. Routine and scheduled breastfeeding sessions
C. Certain sounds or smells associated with the traumatic experience
D. Adequate rest and relaxation during breastfeeding

Correct Answer: C

Rationale:
Sensory stimuli such as specific sounds, smells, or tactile sensations associated with past trauma can trigger PTSD symptoms during breastfeeding.

5. *Defining Trauma*

Question:
What distinguishes trauma from ordinary hardship?

Options:
A. Trauma is always predictable and planned
B. Trauma involves an overwhelming experience that disrupts a person's. sense of safety
C. Trauma only occurs in childhood
D. Trauma is less intense than everyday stress

Correct Answer: B

Rationale:
Trauma is characterised by unpredictability, threat, and a profound disruption of safety, rather than the manageable stressors of everyday life.

6. *Types of Trauma*

Question:
Which of the following correctly lists the categories of trauma discussed in this resource?

Options:
A. Acute, chronic, and developmental
B. Physical, emotional, and spiritual
C. Minor, major, and catastrophic
D. Temporary, permanent, and transitory

Correct Answer: A

Rationale:
Trauma is often conceptualised by duration and timing: acute (single events), chronic (repeated exposure), and developmental (occurring during formative years).

7. *Long-Term Effects of ACEs*

Question:
Which of the following are long-term impacts associated with Adverse Childhood Experiences?

Options:
A. Increased risk for cardiovascular and autoimmune disease
B. Higher likelihood of depression and anxiety
C. Enhanced ability to form secure attachments
D. Both A and B

Correct Answer: D

Rationale:
ACEs are associated with both adverse physical health outcomes and increased rates of mental health conditions. Secure attachment is generally less likely without buffering relationships.

8. *Principles of Trauma-Informed Care*

Question:
What is a core principle of trauma-informed care?

Options:
A. Ignoring past trauma to focus solely on current symptoms
B. Prioritising safety, trust, and empowerment
C. Assuming all patients respond to trauma in the same way
D. Relying primarily on pharmacological treatment

Correct Answer: B

Rationale:
Trauma-informed care centres safety, choice, collaboration, trustworthiness, and empowerment.

9. Neuroscience of Fear

Question:
Which brain structure is commonly referred to as the “fear centre”?

Options:
A. Hippocampus
B. Amygdala
C. Prefrontal cortex
D. Thalamus

Correct Answer: B

Rationale:
The amygdala plays a central role in fear detection and threat processing.

10. Understanding ACT

Question:
In psychotherapy, what does ACT stand for?

Options:
A. Advanced Cognitive Techniques
B. Acceptance and Commitment Therapy
C. Assertive Communication Training
D. Adaptive Coping Techniques

Correct Answer: B

Rationale:
ACT emphasises acceptance of internal experiences and commitment to values-based action.

11. *Holding Space in Therapeutic Relationships*

Question:
Which of the following best describes "holding space"? (Select all that apply.)

Options:
A. Providing immediate solutions
B. Offering empathetic, non-judgemental presence
C. Actively listening and validating emotions
D. Imposing personal beliefs
E. Creating emotional safety

Correct Answer: B, C, E

Rationale:
Holding space involves presence, validation, and safety — not fixing or directing.

12. Benefits of Grounding Techniques

Question:
What are potential benefits of grounding techniques? (Select all that apply.)

Options:
A. Increased dissociation
B. Enhanced emotional regulation
C. Improved focus and attention
D. Reduced depersonalisation
E. Increased panic

Correct Answer: B, C, D

Rationale:
Grounding supports regulation and present-moment awareness.

13. *Reducing Vicarious Trauma*

Question:
What is a proactive strategy to reduce vicarious trauma?

Options:
A. Emotional withdrawal from clients
B. Ignoring personal responses
C. Establishing boundaries and self-care
D. Repeated exposure to traumatic material

Correct Answer: C

Rationale:
Boundaries, supervision, and self-care are protective against secondary trauma.

14. *Considerations for Breastfeeding Decisions*

Question:
When supporting a patient with a trauma history, which factors should be considered in breastfeeding decisions? (Select all that apply.)

Options:
A. Trauma history is irrelevant
B. Emotional comfort and wellbeing
C. Mental health impact
D. Medical considerations
E. Access to support

Correct Answer: B, C, D, E

Rationale:
Trauma-informed feeding decisions integrate emotional, medical, and contextual factors.

APPENDIX B: FURTHER READING AND WEB-BASED RESOURCES

Birth Trauma Resources

Australasian Birth Trauma Association
Website: www.birthtrauma.org.au
Facebook Group: www.facebook.com/groups/birthtrauma.org.au

Books
- How to Heal a Bad Birth – Bruijn & Gould
- Why Birth Trauma Matters – Emma Svanberg

Resources for Past Sexual Trauma

Books
- When Survivors Give Birth – Simkin & Klaus

General Trauma Resources

Books
- The Body Keeps the Score – Bessel van der Kolk
- Trauma Stewardship – Laura van Dernoot Lipsky
- The Happiness Trap – Russ Harris

Online Resources
- This Way Up (self-directed programs for PTSD, anxiety, depression)
- PTSD Coach App
- Headspace (mindfulness and meditation)

Acceptance and Commitment Therapy (ACT) Resources

Books
- ACT Made Simple – Russ Harris
- The Happiness Trap – Russ Harris

Online Resources

- ACT worksheets and summaries: www.actmindfully.com.au
- Videos: "The Struggle Switch", "Doom and Gloom Radio" (Russ Harris)

Training

- ACT Mindfully – 8-week online course

Cognitive Behavioural Therapy (CBT) Resources

Online

- CBT tools and worksheets: www.positivepsychology.com

Grounding Resources

Guided Meditations

- Grounding visualisation (free): Insight Timer – Whole Body Coaching

Visualisation Practices

- Rooted Tree visualisation (free): Insight Timer

Tapping Techniques

- Emotional Freedom Technique (EFT) – YouTube guides

Printable Worksheets

- www.therapistaid.com

Limit-Setting with Toddlers

Children's Books

- Nursies When the Sun Shines
- Booby Moon

Referral Options (Australia)

- Gidget Foundation – www.gidgetfoundation.org.au
- PANDA – www.panda.org.au
- Lifeline – 13 11 14
- Blue Knot Foundation – www.blueknot.org.au
- 1800RESPECT – 1800 737 732

This appendix is intended as a starting point, not an exhaustive list.

APPENDIX C: EXAMPLES OF GROUNDING PRACTICES

Through the Senses

- Barefoot on grass
- Cool or warm water on the face
- Holding textured or comforting objects
- Noticing smells, sounds, sights
- Mindful eating or drinking

Through Movement

- Pressing feet into the ground
- Gentle stretching or swaying
- Walking slowly with awareness
- Rocking or repetitive movement

Through Breath and Awareness

- Slow breathing
- Counting
- Grounding phrases ("I am here", "This is now")

FINAL REFLECTIONS

This work is intended as a layered, clinician-facing resource integrating research, practice, and lived experience. Its purpose is not to prescribe a single approach, but to deepen understanding, sharpen clinical sensitivity, and support reflective, trauma-informed care.

Thank you for the work you do — for the listening, the restraint, the presence, and the courage to sit with complexity. Every time you choose attunement over urgency, and compassion over correction, you contribute to healing that may never be charted — but is nonetheless real.

What you offer is enough.

COMPLETE REFERENCE LIST

1 Association AP. Diagnostic and statistical manual of mental disorders. 5th edition ed. Arlington (VA): American Psychiatric Publishing; 2013.

2 Kimberg L, Wheeler M. Trauma and Trauma-Informed Care. 2019. p. 25–56.

3 Felitti VJ, Anda RF, Nordenberg D, Williamson DF, Spitz AM, Edwards V, et al. Relationship of childhood abuse and household dysfunction to many of the leading causes of death in adults. The Adverse Childhood Experiences (ACE) Study. Am J Prev Med. 1998;14(4):245–58.

4 Kolk vd. The body keeps the score: brain, mind, and body in the healing of trauma. New York: Viking; 2014.

5 Sobel L, O'Rourke-Suchoff D, Holland E, Remis K, Resnick K, Perkins R, et al. Pregnancy and Childbirth After Sexual Trauma: Patient Perspectives and Care Preferences. Obstet Gynecol. 2018;132(6):1461–8.

6 Perera E, Chou S, Cousins N, Mota N, Reynolds K. Women's experiences of trauma, the psychosocial impact and health service needs during the perinatal period. BMC Pregnancy Childbirth. 2023;23(1):197.

7 Callanan F, Bradshaw C, Tuohy T, Noonan M, Murphy S, Grealish A. An integrative review of how midwives are screening and assessing for trauma in women within perinatal services. PLoS One. 2025;20(7):e0327253.

8 Kendall-Tackett K, Cong Z, Hale TW. Depression, sleep quality, and maternal well-being in postpartum women with a history of sexual assault: a comparison of breastfeeding, mixed-feeding, and formula-feeding mothers. Breastfeed Med. 2013;8(1):16–22.

9 Miller ES, Fleming O, Ekpe EE, Grobman WA, Heard-Garris N. Association Between Adverse Childhood Experiences and Adverse Pregnancy Outcomes. Obstet Gynecol. 2021;138(5):770–6.

10 Mamun A, Biswas T, Scott J, Sly PD, McIntyre HD, Thorpe K, et al. Adverse childhood experiences, the risk of pregnancy complications and adverse pregnancy outcomes: a systematic review and meta-analysis. BMJ Open. 2023;13(8):e063826.

11 Swedo EA, D'Angelo DV, Fasula AM, Clayton HB, Ports KA. Associations of Adverse Childhood Experiences With Pregnancy and Infant Health. Am J Prev Med. 2023;64(4):512–24.

12 Roubinov DS, Luecken LJ, Curci SG, Somers JA, Winstone LK. A prenatal programming perspective on the intergenerational transmission of maternal adverse childhood experiences to offspring health problems. Am Psychol. 2021;76(2):337–49.

13 Racine N, Plamondon A, Madigan S, McDonald S, Tough S. Maternal Adverse Childhood Experiences and Infant Development. Pediatrics. 2018;141(4).

14 Johnson S, Kasparian NA, Cullum AS, Flanagan T, Ponting C, Kowalewski L, et al. Addressing Adverse Childhood and Adult Experiences During Prenatal Care. Obstet Gynecol. 2023;141(6):1072–87.

15 Borg LE, Alhusen JL. A Review of Factors that Serve to Protect Pregnant and Post-partum Women from Negative Outcomes Associated with Adverse Childhood Experiences. Matern Child Health J. 2023;27(9):1503–17.

16 Isobel S. Trauma and the perinatal period: A review of the theory and practice of trauma-sensitive interactions for nurses and midwives. Nurs Open. 2023;10(12):7585–95.

17 Sperlich M, Seng JS, Li Y, Taylor J, Bradbury-Jones C. Integrating Trauma-Informed Care Into Maternity Care Practice: Conceptual and Practical Issues. J Midwifery Womens Health. 2017;62(6):661–72.

18 Kezelman C, Stavropoulos P. Practice guidelines for treatment of complex trauma and trauma-informed care. Sydney: Blue Knot Foundation; 2012.

19 Purkiewicz A, Regin KJ, Pietrzak-Fiećko R. Breastfeeding in the Context of Trauma and Previous Psychological Experiences: A Narrative Review. Nutrients. 2026;18(3).

20 Martini J, Asselmann E, Weidner K, Knappe S, Rosendahl J, Garthus-Niegel S. Prospective Associations of Lifetime Post-traumatic Stress Disorder and Birth-Related Traumatization With Maternal and Infant Outcomes. Front Psychiatry. 2022;13:842410.

21 Channell Doig A, Jasczynski M, Fleishman JL, Aparicio EM. Breastfeeding Among Mothers Who Have Experienced Childhood Maltreatment: A Review. J Hum Lact. 2020;36(4):710–22.

22 Cavallé-Abasolo E, Dikmen-Yildiz P, Gómez-Gómez I, Barros-Martins L, Motrico E. Impact of Traumatic Childbirth and Birth-Related Posttraumatic Stress Disorder on Breastfeeding Outcomes: A Systematic Review of Longitudinal and Cohort Studies. Birth. 2025;52(4):553–71.

23 Beery AK, Jackson B, Halstead E, Windorski SM, Nnodim-Amadi C, Upin E. Acute decrease in mothers' cortisol following nursing and milk expression. Horm Behav. 2023;153:105387.

24 Wheeler A, Sweeting F, Mayers A, Brown A, Farrington S. Improving perinatal mental health outcomes: The role of support in assisting breastfeeding experiences following birth trauma. Midwifery. 2026;152:104668.

25 Uvnäs Moberg K, Ekström-Bergström A, Buckley S, Massarotti C, Pajalic Z, Luegmair K, et al. Maternal plasma levels of oxytocin during breastfeeding-A systematic review. PLoS One. 2020;15(8):e0235806.

26 Engel S, Klusmann H, Laufer S, Pfeifer AC, Ditzen B, van Zuiden M, et al. Trauma exposure, posttraumatic stress disorder and oxytocin: A meta-analytic investigation of endogenous concentrations and receptor genotype. Neurosci Biobehav Rev. 2019;107:560–601.

27 Witteveen AB, Stramrood CAI, Henrichs J, Flanagan JC, van Pampus MG, Olff M. The oxytocinergic system in PTSD following traumatic childbirth: endogenous and exogenous oxytocin in the peripartum period. Arch Womens Ment Health. 2020;23(3):317–29.

28 Sharma SR, Gonda X, Dome P, Tarazi FI. What's Love Got to do with it: Role of oxytocin in trauma, attachment and resilience. Pharmacol Ther. 2020;214:107602.

29 Donadon MF, Martin-Santos R, Osório FL. The Associations Between Oxytocin and Trauma in Humans: A Systematic Review. Front Pharmacol. 2018;9:154.

30 Dewey KG. Maternal and fetal stress are associated with impaired lactogenesis in humans. J Nutr. 2001;131(11):3012s–5s.

31 Karakoyunlu Ö, Ejder Apay S, Gürol A. The effect of pain, stress, and cortisol during labor on breastfeeding success. Dev Psychobiol. 2019;61(7):979–87.

32 Matyas M, Apanasewicz A, Krzystek-Korpacka M, Jamrozik N, Cierniak A, Babiszewska-Aksamit M, et al. The association between maternal stress and human milk concentrations of cortisol and prolactin. Sci Rep. 2024;14(1):28115.

33 Bengtson L, Aubuchon-Endsley NL. Prenatal depression moderates the relationship between maternal trauma exposure and cortisol production and predicts breastfeeding behavior. Women Health. 2023;63(5):334–45.

34 Wood K, Van Esterik P. Infant feeding experiences of women who were sexually abused in childhood. Can Fam Physician. 2010;56(4):e136–41.

35 Jones KA, Freijah I, Brennan SE, McKenzie JE, Bright TM, Fiolet R, et al. Interventions from pregnancy to two years after birth for parents experiencing complex post-traumatic stress disorder and/or with childhood experience of maltreatment. Cochrane Database Syst Rev. 2023;5(5):Cd014874.

36 Elfgen C, Hagenbuch N, Görres G, Block E, Leeners B. Breastfeeding in Women Having Experienced Childhood Sexual Abuse. J Hum Lact. 2017;33(1):119–27.

37 Caring for Patients Who Have Experienced Trauma: ACOG Committee Opinion, Number 825. Obstetrics & Gynecology. 2021;137(4):e94–e9.

38 Prentice JC, Lu MC, Lange L, Halfon N. The association between reported childhood sexual abuse and breastfeeding initiation. J Hum Lact. 2002;18(3):219–26.

39 Sørbø MF, Lukasse M, Brantsæter AL, Grimstad H. Past and recent abuse is associated with early cessation of breast feeding: results from a large prospective cohort in Norway. BMJ Open. 2015;5(12):e009240.

40 Coles J, Anderson A, Loxton D. Breastfeeding Duration after Childhood Sexual Abuse: An Australian Cohort Study. J Hum Lact. 2016;32(3):Np28–35.

41 Ukah UV, Adu PA, De Silva DA, von Dadelszen P. The Impact of a History of Adverse Childhood Experiences on Breastfeeding Initiation and Exclusivity: Findings from a National Population Health Survey. Breastfeed Med. 2016;11:544–50.

42 McCloskey RJ, Pei F. Associations Between Mothers' Adverse Childhood Experiences, Material Hardship, and Breastfeeding Challenges in the United States. J Hum Lact. 2022;38(4):651–60.

43 Watson C, Wei J, Varnado N, Rios N, Flanagan T, Alabaster A, et al. Adverse Childhood Experiences and Early and Continued Breastfeeding: Findings from an Integrated Health Care Delivery System. J Womens Health (Larchmt). 2021;30(3):367–76.

44 Do HP, Vo TV, Murray L, Baker PRA, Murray A, Valdebenito S, et al. The influence of childhood abuse and prenatal intimate partner violence on childbirth experiences and breastfeeding outcomes. Child Abuse Negl. 2022;131:105743.

45 Barriers to Breastfeeding: Supporting Initiation and Continuation of Breastfeeding: ACOG Committee Opinion, Number 821. Obstetrics & Gynecology. 2021;137(2):e54–e62.

46 Forkey H, Szilagyi M, Kelly ET, Duffee J. Trauma-Informed Care. Pediatrics. 2021;148(2).

47 Wheeler A, Sweeting F, Mayers A, Brown A, Farrington S. The Positive Cycle of Breastfeeding-Mental Health Outcomes of Breastfeeding Mothers Following Birth Trauma. Healthcare (Basel). 2025;13(6).

48 Australia BT. What is birth trauma? n.d. [Birth Trauma Australia]. Available from: https://birthtrauma.org.au/what-is-birth-trauma/.

49 Dekel S, Stuebe C, Dishy G. Childbirth Induced Posttraumatic Stress Syndrome: A Systematic Review of Prevalence and Risk Factors. Front Psychol. 2017;8:560.

50 Wosu AC, Gelaye B, Williams MA. History of childhood sexual abuse and risk of prenatal and postpartum depression or depressive symptoms: an epidemiologic review. Arch Womens Ment Health. 2015;18(5):659–71.

51 Gordon J, Hunter A, Callanan F, Kiely C, Grealish A. An Integrative Review Exploring Womens' Experiences of Retraumatization Within Perinatal Services. J Midwifery Womens Health. 2025;70(1):32–49.

52 Pidd D, Newton M, Wilson I, East C. Optimising maternity care for a subsequent pregnancy after a psychologically traumatic birth: A scoping review. Women Birth. 2023;36(5):e471–e80.

53 Grekin R, O'Hara MW. Prevalence and risk factors of postpartum posttraumatic stress disorder: a meta-analysis. Clin Psychol Rev. 2014;34(5):389–401.

54 Yildiz PD, Ayers S, Phillips L. The prevalence of posttraumatic stress disorder in pregnancy and after birth: A systematic review and meta-analysis. J Affect Disord. 2017;208:634–45.

55 McEvoy PM, Grove R, Slade T. Epidemiology of anxiety disorders in the Australian general population: findings of the 2007 Australian National Survey of Mental Health and Wellbeing. Aust N Z J Psychiatry. 2011;45(11):957–67.

56 Beck CT, Watson S. Impact of birth trauma on breast-feeding: a tale of two pathways. Nurs Res. 2008;57(4):228–36.

57 Davis AMB, Sclafani V. Birth Experiences, Breastfeeding, and the Mother-Child Relationship: Evidence from a Large Sample of Mothers. Can J Nurs Res. 2022;54(4):518–29.

58 Mersky JP, Lee CP. Adverse childhood experiences and poor birth outcomes in a diverse, low-income sample. BMC Pregnancy Childbirth. 2019;19(1):387.

59 Nesari M, Olson JK, Vandermeer B, Slater L, Olson DM. Does a maternal history of abuse before pregnancy affect pregnancy outcomes? A systematic review with meta-analysis. BMC Pregnancy Childbirth. 2018;18(1):404.

60 Kern A, Khoury B, Frederickson A, Langevin R. The associations between childhood maltreatment and pregnancy complications: A systematic review and meta-analysis. J Psychosom Res. 2022;160:110985.

61 Seng JS, Low LK, Sperlich M, Ronis DL, Liberzon I. Prevalence, trauma history, and risk for posttraumatic stress disorder among nulliparous women in maternity care. Obstet Gynecol. 2009;114(4):839–47.

62 Malouf R, Harrison S, Burton HAL, Gale C, Stein A, Franck LS, et al. Prevalence of anxiety and post-traumatic stress (PTS) among the parents of babies admitted to neonatal units: A systematic review and meta-analysis. EClinicalMedicine. 2022;43:101233.

63 Horan H, Ryu J, Stone J, Thurston L. Healing trauma with interprofessional collaboration and trauma-informed perinatal care: A qualitative case study. Birth. 2023;50(3):525–34.

64 Sokou R, Parastatidou S, Ioakeimidis G, Tavoulari EF, Makrogianni A, Isaakidou E, et al. Breastfeeding in Neonates Admitted to an NICU: 18-Month Follow-Up. Nutrients. 2022;14(18).

65 Organization WH. Infant and young child feeding. World Health Organisation; 2023.

66 Kendall-Tackett K. Psychological Trauma and Breastfeeding: What We Know So Far. Medical Research Archives. 2022;10.

67 Moog NK, Buss C, Entringer S, Shahbaba B, Gillen DL, Hobel CJ, et al. Maternal Exposure to Childhood Trauma Is Associated During Pregnancy With Placental-Fetal Stress Physiology. Biol Psychiatry. 2016;79(10):831–9.

68 Beck CT, Watson S. Subsequent childbirth after a previous traumatic birth. Nurs Res. 2010;59(4):241–9.

69 COPE. Mental health care in the perinatal period: Australian clinical practice guideline. Melbourne: Centre of Perinatal Excellence (COPE); 2023.

70 Strathearn L, Mamun AA, Najman JM, O'Callaghan MJ. Does breastfeeding protect against substantiated child abuse and neglect? A 15-year cohort study. Pediatrics. 2009;123(2):483–93.

71 White A, Saxer K, Raja S, Hall SL. A Trauma-informed Approach to Postpartum Care. Clin Obstet Gynecol. 2022;65(3):550–62.

72 SAMHSA. SAMHSA's Concept of Trauma and Guidance for a Trauma-Informed Approach. Rockville, MD; 2014. Report No.: (SMA) 14-4884.

73 Levine PA. In an Unspoken Voice: How the Body Releases Trauma and Restores Goodness. Berkeley: North Atlantic Books; 2010.

74 Nichols MP, Straus MB. The Lost Art of Listening: How Learning to Listen Can Improve Relationships. 3rd ed. New York: Guilford Press; 2021.

75 van der Kolk B. The Body Keeps the Score: Brain, Mind, and Body in the Healing of Trauma. New York: Viking; 2014.

76 van der Kolk BA. Clinical implications of neuroscience research in PTSD. Ann N Y Acad Sci. 2006;1071:277–93.

77 Whitley J, Wouk K, Bauer AE, Grewen K, Gottfredson NC, Meltzer-Brody S, et al. Oxytocin during breastfeeding and maternal mood symptoms. Psychoneuroendocrinology. 2020;113:104581.

78 Porges S. The Polyvagal Theory. New York: Norton.

79 Harris R. ACT Made Simple. 2nd ed. Oakland, CA: New Harbinger Publications; 2025.

80 Winnicott DW. Transitional objects and transitional phenomena; a study of the first not-me possession. Int J Psychoanal. 1953;34(2):89–97.

81 Beck CT. Birth trauma: in the eye of the beholder. Nurs Res. 2004;53(1):28–35.

82 Dennis CL. Peer support within a health care context: a concept analysis. Int J Nurs Stud. 2003;40(3):321–32.

83 Ravi A, Gorelick J, Pal H. Identifying and Addressing Vicarious Trauma. Am Fam Physician. 2021;103(9):570-2.

84 Forkey H, Szilagyi M, Kelly ET, Duffee J, THE COUNCIL ON FOSTER CARE A, KINSHIP CARE COCP, COUNCIL ON CHILD ABUSE, et al. Trauma-Informed Care. Pediatrics. 2021;148(2).

85 Rogers CR. The necessary and sufficient conditions of therapeutic personality change. 1957. J Consult Clin Psychol. 1992;60(6):827–32.

www.ingramcontent.com/pod-product-compliance
Lightning Source LLC
LaVergne TN
LVHW022217200926
848481LV00006B/1999

* 9 7 8 1 7 6 4 3 1 8 3 2 7 *